PAIN BANISHMENT

Don't manage your pain
Banish it completely!

Even when nothing else works...

Get Your Life Back with a Non-invasive Treatment for RSD/ CRPS, Neuropathy, Fibromyalgia, and Other Chronic Pain

Book One in the *Pain Banishment* Series

NationWide Publishers

Dr. Donald Rhodes and Patricia Boeckman

Visit Dr. Rhodes' website at:

www.paindefeat.com

For additional copies of this book, go to:

PainBanishment.com **OR** email: PainBanishment@yahoo.com

Many grateful patients have written glowing letters of gratitude to Dr. Donald Rhodes to thank him for defeating their pain, restoring their health, and even saving their life. He has gathered their writings in a binder and posted many of them on the bulletin board in his office.

I join that group of patients with this book. It is my thank you letter to Dr. Rhodes.
~ *Patricia Boeckman*

Thanks to my husband, writer Charles Boeckman, for editorial guidance in the production of this book. His life-time of writing experience was invaluable.

I am grateful to my wonderful daughter, Sharla Wilkins, for her help with this book and especially for her input on the back cover copy, which reflects her insight and astute eye for verbal clarity.

I want to give special recognition to Dusty White for making this book cover possible.

Special thanks to Tamara, who worked so willingly to facilitate the publication of this book. Not only did she proofread, but she also tirelessly promoted this book's message to help those in pain, even while still suffering before her recovery was complete. I was sure she would help. That's the kind of person she is, and I know her well.

My appreciation goes to graphic illustrator Mary Martin, who contributed graphics for this book; to Laurene Gatlin for help with proofreading; to writer and friend Maury Breecher for editorial input; to Irene Volle for suggested changes; to Julie Tirpak for pointing out technical errors: and to my Mother, Juanita Bird, for her lifetime of dedication to helping others, including her invaluable support for this work. I am grateful to all the many people who proofread this book and offered suggestions.

Table of Contents

Preface

Part One—The Miracle Man

Part Two—Miracle Remissions

Part Three—Clinical and Scholarly Research

Appendix

This book, like all my writing, is dedicated to my beloved husband,
Charles Boeckman.

Preface

Elliot T. Udell, D.P.M.

Fellow of the American College of Podiatric Medicine
Diplomat of the American Academy of Pain Management
Diplomat of the American College of Foot and Ankle Orthopedists and Pod. Med.
Hicksville, New York

I have had the great honor of studying under Dr. Donald Rhodes. I studied at his office in Corpus Christi, Texas, where I observed him caring for numerous patients. I also presented him with select cases I was treating at my home office, and I gladly received his expert opinion on how to best medically manage these cases.

Dr. Rhodes is an authority on the treatment of Complex Regional Pain Syndrome, better known as Reflex Sympathetic Dystrophy Syndrome. This condition that affects millions of Americans causes severe pain and disability. In its early stages it presents with debilitating pain, and in later stages it interferes with the person's ability to properly ambulate. The symptoms are so severe that they incapacitate the affected individual, interfering with any and every aspect of his or her life. Affected people not only cannot enjoy their lives but also in most cases cannot work for a living.

Dr. Rhodes has developed a system of intense electro-stimulation, which if used properly, can rapidly put RSDS into remission. I met patients at his office who initially could not move without the use of a cane, walker, or wheel chair. Within 15 days of intense therapy, these patients were able to walk without the use of assisting devices and they were pain free.

Treatments that are being employed by other doctors for the treatment of RSDS include spinal injections, massive doses of narcotic analgesics, spinal implants of analgesic pumps, stimulators, or even surgical ablation of the sympathetic ganglia. All of these latter treatments are expensive, give temporary relief, and carry a degree of medical risk. Dr. Rhodes' methods not only bring relief to suffering patients but they do not economically overburden the already financially stressed health care system in this country. They are also safe.

There was an earlier problem with having all physicians nationwide use Dr. Rhodes' methods due to many different modalities that had to be employed. However, Dr. Rhodes developed a single machine that combines all the modalities he originally used in the treatment of RSD. This unit, which is user friendly, will enable doctors from all over the country and even from all over the world to effectively and economically treat and manage this dreadful condition.

Dr. Rhodes has been a partner to any doctor anywhere who seeks his help in managing patients with Complex Regional Pain Syndrome. Several times a year I communicate with him about patients who need help and he has always helped out. He is not only a genius of a doctor but his heart is in the right place when it comes to taking care of fellow human beings.

Because so many people are suffering and physicians from all over are clamoring for such a modality, anything that can be done to rapidly render this device in the hands of practicing doctors will be a blessing to millions of suffering men, women, and children.

"If I hadn't found Dr. Rhodes, I would have killed myself. Life with that kind of pain was no longer worth living. I would have raised my kids, and then that would have been it for me."

Pat

PART ONE—THE MIRACLE MAN

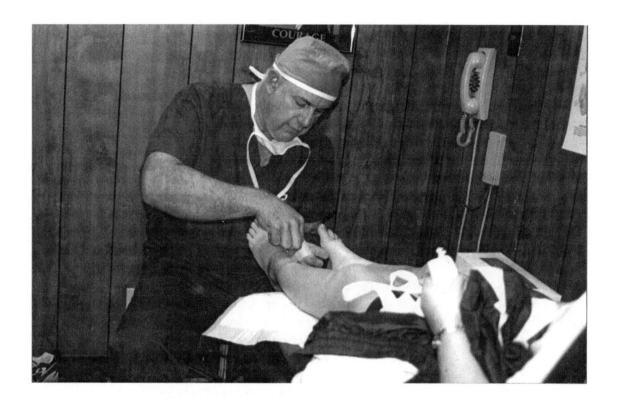

CHAPTER ONE

TAPPED ON THE SHOULDER BY FATE

What event first led me into pain banishment?

In 1992 when I poised my scalpel over the foot of my latest surgery patient, Maria, I had no idea that her outcome would dramatically alter the course of my medical career and my life.

A board certified podiatric surgeon, I had spent approximately twenty years doing foot surgery. I performed twenty to forty surgeries a week with excellent results. Although I saw patients with neuropathy, a type of unrelenting nerve pain, I didn't primarily deal with that condition.

However, in 1992, everything changed when I operated on Maria's foot. She had a double wedge osteotomy, a procedure involving multiple bone cutting surgery. Her recovery required a non-weight bearing cast. After surgery or injuries, patients sometimes develop a kind of Super Bowl of neuropathy called Reflex Sympathetic Dystrophy Syndrome, or RSDS. It is also shortened to RSD. A more recent name for it is Complex Regional Pain Syndrome, or CRPS. The name change resulted from a new understanding of this disease. It was once thought to be confined to a specific part of the body, usually an extremity. However, when doctors began to learn that RSD can spread to other parts of the body and cause pain in multiple locations, the name was updated to CRPS to reflect the widespread nature of the malady in many patients.

In my medical practice, I prescribed a lot of post-operative physical therapy, and I think that's why my patients didn't develop chronic pain. However, because of Maria's cast, I couldn't prescribe the usual amount of such therapy, and that led to an unexpected, dreadful outcome. She developed RSD. Although it can take hold in any part of the body, it commonly develops in an extremity, often in the foot. It is characterized by searing, excruciating pain, often numbness, and sometimes atrophy. In severe cases, when it strikes, the foot can suddenly swell to twice its normal size and measure fifteen degrees colder than the other foot. The

OTHER SYMPTOMS OF RSD:
1. Inflammation
2. Muscle twitches
3. Insomnia
4. Depression
5. Memory loss
6. Irritability
7. Fatigue
8. Grooved, brittle nails
9. Loss of bone density

skin in the affected area can change color, sometimes to a shiny, deep purple. A person with RSD suffers unremitting pain. It's not like any normal pain you've ever experienced. It feels like a gigantic, fiery screw turning and twisting down with a kind of tearing sensation. The pain persists 24 hours a day, seven days a week, with no breaks. It is sheer, constant agony. That much I knew. Only later did I learn the full scope of this condition.

But back to Maria. When her pain from the operation persisted and even worsened, I carefully examined her foot. No definitive test for RSD existed. Diagnosis depended on the skill of the doctor to recognize the signs and symptoms, which I did.

"It looks like you have RSD," I told Maria. "I'm not an expert in this. Let me find someone who is and who's getting good results after treatment."

What I learned was discouraging, at best. The doctors I called consistently reported that nobody was getting good results managing RSD. They said the condition usually became chronic and had no specific treatment. I decided to check out the medical literature. I found that the condition had been diagnosed in injured soldiers as far back as the Civil War. However, in spite of its long tenure on record, scant information existed about how to fix the problem. Everything dealt with describing and diagnosing the stages of RSD based on symptoms. Nobody got better.

When I told Maria the bad news, she looked me in the eyes and said, "You're the smartest doctor I know, so I guess you're going to have to figure out how to treat it."

Her comment touched me deeply. I had to do something. Maybe it was fate tapping on my shoulder. Perhaps it was the challenge of figuring out the answer to the puzzle of RSD in order to help Maria, whose condition was worsening. Or I could have been so ignorant of the enormity of the task that I thought I'd find some rather simple approach to Maria's problem that would work. If so, I'd be back at the operating table in short order. Or so I assumed.

Whatever motivated me, I felt driven. I set out on a quest of intense research. I was overwhelmed by what I learned.

I was astonished at the extent of suffering due to pain.

I found that 70 to 80 million Americans suffer from chronic pain. At its simplest level, chronic pain means hurting that lasts longer than it should. For example, if you bump your elbow on a corner, it shouldn't still hurt three months later. If it does, or if the pain worsens for no apparent reason, something is definitely wrong. Something is also definitely wrong when chronic pain results from an illness, such as diabetes. About half of all diabetics develop peripheral neuropathy, which usually begins with tingling in the feet. It escalates into burning pain and spreads up the legs.

At its worst, chronic pain can develop into RSD. When that happens, life becomes a nightmare. In addition to the wracking, burning pain, patients often become highly sensitized to any touch, so that even air blowing across the affected area can be torture. They can feel as if they're on fire. Muscle spasms, lesions that won't heal, swelling, muscle atrophy, tremors, insomnia, depression, brain fog, overwhelming fatigue, feelings of weakness, and ear buzzing are some common additional symptoms. Life as they have known it ends.

Unfortunately, many RSD patients are told their symptoms are all in their head.

"The doctors who saw my daughter didn't believe she was hurting. Her crying, her arm turning purple, none of that convinced them she wasn't putting on. They repeatedly told me she was imagining the pain." Patient's mother.

These patients often see a series of doctors before receiving a correct diagnosis. Their treatment options traditionally range from operations, to pain killers, nerve blocks, implantation of nerve stimulators, narcotics, morphine pumps, physical therapy and exercise, diet, mental imaging, etc. Some of these methods make the patient worse. Some leave the sufferer in a perpetual mental fog. The typical objective has been pain *management*, which is a euphemism for learning to live with a certain level of pain. My objective was, and is, pain *banishment*.

I believe pain management is a cop out. A famous quote says, "In war, there is no prize for second place. You're merely the first place loser." The same can be said for battling pain. If you can't eliminate it entirely, you've actually lost the battle. Even pain rated in the mid-range of intensity or lower can diminish your quality of life. For instance, if you like to go window shopping at the mall, you may stay home instead because of constant discomfort. After a time, you reach a point where you literally can't go anymore. This deterioration is explained by a law I learned in medical school. It says that physical or physiological structures which have stress applied grow stronger. However, the converse is also true. That is, the same structures with no stress applied grow weaker. So when you can't comfortably go to the mall, then don't go to the mall, eventually you physically can't go to the mall. What's keeping you home isn't just the pain. It's that your physical and emotional structures have become weak.

In addition to the personal toll, chronic pain costs around $100 billion dollars each year in medical expenses, lost income, and absence from work. Its drain on the U.S. economy eclipses any other chronic condition, including diabetes, hypertension, and heart disease. It also can batter the entire family emotionally and financially as their lives constantly revolve around attempts to find a palliative for the person in pain. A case in point is my patient I call the Million Dollar Man. Felled by a knee injury that turned into RSD and spread through his body, he spent seven years and had incurred over a million dollars in insurance claims while looking in vain for relief before he learned about me. You'll read his story in his own words later in this book.

Finally, according to a pain specialist, "Pain can kill. It can kill the spirit, vitality, and the will to live."

So we're not talking about a benign condition. Chronic pain treacherously devastates because it often has not been taken as a serious threat to health and even today lacks a coordinated, successful approach to treatment.

My research led me into unexpected terrain.

Given what I already knew plus what I learned about the RSD through research, I set out to devise a treatment for Maria. I would love to say it was flashes of brilliance that led me to the discoveries that set me off in the right direction. The truth is, it was mainly hard work. I spent countless hours pouring over medical research, studying, and gathering bits and pieces of scattered information that I put together to devise a treatment that might work. It involved educating myself in ways I'd never imagined.

I found studies that pointed me in particular directions. Specifically, I needed to forget drugs, surgeries, exercise, and all the rest, because those approaches addressed only symptoms. Instead I needed to focus on some type of electrical stimulation of the sympathetic nervous system, which would treat the actual underlying cause of pain. That meant I needed some sort of machine. The key was to start with existing electrical stimulation modalities and reconfigure them in a new way. That was an unexpected challenge, to develop a unique approach that worked differently from everything else available. A treatment that, instead of camouflaging symptoms, could actually treat the underlying cause of chronic pain.

So that's what I did. I cobbled together a rather primitive system, compared to what I later developed, and treated Maria. It took a while, but as she improved, she spread the word to her friends. They started coming into my office with migraine headaches, jaw pain, and peripheral neuropathy. I treated them all, and they improved right along with Maria. In fact, when her treatments ended, she left my office with no more RSD symptoms and returned to wearing high heels. Since then, I have mainly treated chronic pain and have continued research and clinical studies to find better, faster ways to banish it.

What I have learned in the process has been truly amazing.

HIGHLIGHTS FROM CHAPTER 1

1. Chronic pain affects 70 to 80 million Americans.
2. Chronic pain costs around $100 billion a year in medical expenses, lost income, and absence from work.
3. In 1992, I had a patient with RSD, a severe form of chronic pain.
4. I conducted research on RSD, which was considered untreatable, and devised a treatment.
5. My RSD patient recovered, and I embarked on a crusade to banish chronic pain.

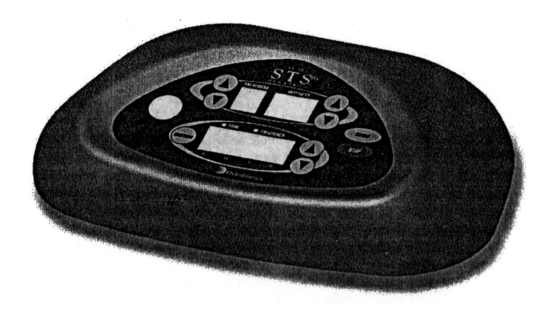

CHAPTER TWO

A GUNSLINGER NO MORE

**Why my medical specialty has been an advantage in developing
a unique pain treatment.**

Since as a podiatrist I am licensed to treat feet, people find it strange that I could also be a pain specialist. But being a podiatrist makes me uniquely qualified for what I do.

Pain results from nerve impulses. The feet are resplendent with nerve endings that affect other parts of the body. Many acupuncture points are found on them. Since my specialty is the ankle and below, I know a great deal about the feet and their nerves, and I have free rein to use any therapies on them I believe will benefit the patient.

When I set out to help my patient Maria, my research indicated that malfunction of the nerves created the pain of RSD and that specific types of electrical stimulation seemed likely to restore the nerve to normal. So the procedure I first developed involved attaching electrodes to areas of specific nerve endings on Maria's feet, the site of her pain. The electrodes were alternately connected by wires to a variety of machines that sent electrical impulses through the nerves. It was trial and error followed by continuing research and refinement.

After Maria recovered, I found from working on other patients that, to make the nerves respond better, I needed to stimulate them over longer distances than just from the toe to the ankle. I was running out of enough foot to do that. Then, in one brief moment of insight, I realized that I could use the patient's other foot, which was connected by nerves that run through the spine. Stimulating a nerve from one foot through the spine and all the way to the other foot provided a tremendously long run.

The first patient on whom I hooked up both feet began to recover faster. So I began adding more machines and electrodes. Other doctors who were licensed to treat the entire body provided support by working with me so we could place electrodes on the legs, arms, and hands, allowing me to treat RSD in all parts of the body. I continued to make long runs through the nerves by sending the electrical impulses from one hand to the other, one arm to the other, or one leg to the other.

I had to make a radical change in my approach to treating chronic pain.

Additional research helped me discover the best electrical frequencies and other technicalities involved with the electrical stimulation to get better results. I added more and more refinements until, after a few years, my patients looked like a stereo system. They were hooked up to six different machines all at once and had 24 electrical pads on them at the same time. Keep in mind, these were long term, chronic pain patients who had been treated by other doctors without success. Most of them had endured excruciating pain for years. Usually, they heard about me through word of mouth from one of my patients and came to me as their last hope. But everybody was improving.

Then a doctor from a pain clinic in Houston came down for a visit. He'd seen some of my patients, and he wanted to know what I was doing that he wasn't doing. He took one look at my set up and said, "This is far too complex. You have to reduce this to one machine. Pick out the primary thing you're doing and go with that. You have to simplify this so it can spread across the United States and across the world."

I gave what that doctor said a lot of thought. I conducted more extensive research and worked long and hard to design the single, unique STS® (Sympathetic Treatment System) machine and modalities that I use today.

My foray into pain banishment without cutting, sawing, or stitching completely transformed my practice. Before my transformation, I was like other modern surgeons whose approach resembles that of the old-fashioned gunslinger from the Wild West. As he reached for his pistol, the gunslinger's answer to every situation was, "Yes, Ma'am. We can fix the problem with hot lead." Likewise, as today's surgeon reaches for his scalpel, he says, "Yes. We can fix the problem with a fifteen blade." Because of their medical training and years of performing surgery, surgeons believe that if you have a problem, an operation is the answer. I thought that, too, before I found a better way.

How did a surgeon, whose daughter developed RSD, react to my non-invasive, drug-free treatment for his offspring?

Dr. Roy Mathews also held tightly to confidence in his medical training--until his own daughter fell into the abyss of unbearable pain for which he and her treating neurologist could find no solutions.

He wrote me this letter in 1999 after I treated her:

Dear Dr. Rhodes:

First let me say thanks for directing the therapy which has restored my daughter to health. As you recall, Kristal was referred to you with acute Reflex Sympathetic Dystrophy (RSD) involving the right shoulder, arm and hand. As a physician, I left medical school thinking that if a medical problem couldn't be treated with a sharp knife, a pill or potion, or psychological counseling, chances are it couldn't be resolved. I watched as my daughter lay in a hospital bed for five days receiving orthodox therapy: narcotics for pain every two hours, multiple injections, IV fluids, sympathetic ganglion blocks, physical ther-

apy, etc., with no apparent benefit. After the fifth day, the neurologist managing her case confided to me that his plan of therapy was not working and that I should consider another option.

Upon explaining to me that there was an alternate form of therapy available, he referred me to your clinic. With my clinical background, I admit I was somewhat skeptical about any treatment of which I had no knowledge or information and viewed any therapy that deviated from main stream medicine with a somewhat jaundiced eye. However, I felt like a drowning man grasping for a straw. I found that straw at your clinic. As you examined my daughter and explained to me your finding, I was impressed with your knowledge of anatomy and pathophysiology. When you told me you could help my daughter and outlined your planned course of therapy, I was encouraged but remained somewhat skeptical.

As we left your office after the first treatment and headed for the hotel, my daughter said, "Dad, I feel funny." I said, "Are you dizzy, nauseated or feel weak?" No, "just feel funny." I took her to her room, put her to bed, and gave her a mild sedative in hopes that she could get some rest. Sir, when she awoke some 12 hours later, she was pain free, the edema in her arm had diminished, the cyanosis in her hand was absent and she had full range of motion of the limb. Now I have never been one to believe much in miracles, but this comes close to qualifying. Thank God, she has been pain free since the initial treatment and has remained so to date.

She has now returned to college to complete her final semester in nursing school. She is completely symptom free. Before, she was depressed, lost interest in her career and in constant pain. She is now optimistic, energetic, pain free, eager to complete her studies and embark upon a new career. You have certainly opened my eyes to a whole new field of medical therapy which I did not know existed. Thanks to you and your supportive, professional and competent staff. You were a Godsend to me and my family. God bless you and yours.

Sincerely,
Dr. Roy Mathews

Kristal completed nursing school and became a pediatric nurse.

The treatment I designed for Maria in 1992 underwent continuous upgrades, so that Kristal in 1999 fell heir to more advanced therapies. Patients now and in the future will benefit from further refinements. That's what medicine is all about: continuously better treatments, continuously better results. But to take advantage of those better treatments and better results, the medical community and patients have to know what is available and how effective it is. In regard to treating chronic pain, this book is one step in that direction.

HIGHLIGHTS FROM CHAPTER 2

1. Pain results from nerve impulses.
2. As a podiatrist, I am uniquely qualified to treat chronic pain because of my expertise in the physiology of the feet, which are resplendent with nerve endings that affect other parts of the body.
3. I discovered that electrically stimulating nerves from one side of the body to the other enhanced pain recovery.
4. I combined many treatment machines into one with unique characteristics.
5. My treatment methods continue to evolve.

"After years of failed treatments and being bed-ridden for a year as I continued to dereriorate, I was dying. At almost the last minute, someone discovered Dr. Rhodes. Three weeks after he began treating me, I walked out of his office restored to health."

Colleen

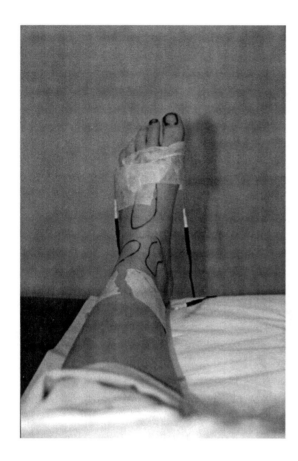 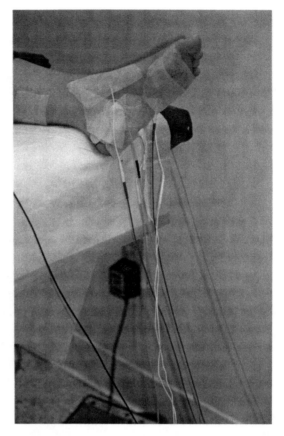

CHAPTER THREE

THE GOOD GUYS AND THE BAD GUYS

Why do I treat every tiny pain, no matter how insignificant it seems to the patient?

I learned a great deal from my patients as I worked to improve my treatments and achieve better results. A major tenet I observed over the years was that patients' pain didn't start to abate until it diminished all over their body. That is, if a patient had a source of pain anywhere that I didn't treat, the patient also failed to recover from the main source of pain. It didn't matter whether their primary pain was in the foot. If they also had migraine headaches, the foot of a chronic pain sufferer was never going to get 100 percent better so long as they had those migraines.

> *"With a black marker, I circled the painful spots on my feet. Dr. Rhodes used his machine and knocked out the painful spots, one by one." Morgan.*

I finally ran across a study that explained this phenomenon. Any kind of chronic nerve pain results from insufficient oxygen to the nerve. Mechanical, surgical, or disease-induced oxygen deprivation to the nerve results in reduced nerve conduction. Increasing the oxygen flow to the nerve normalizes nerve conduction. In simple terms, less oxygen flow to the nerve results in pain. Normal oxygen flow stops pain.

You can check this out yourself. You can wrap a rubber band snugly around your finger, as most kids have done in middle school to see who could endure the discomfort the longest. How long before you feel pain? Probably less than three minutes. You can't cut off circulation from any part of your body for any length of time without running into trouble. That's because when you cut off the blood supply, you also cut off the oxygen.

What is myelin and why is it important?

My treatment resolves pain caused by lack of oxygen. If you lack oxygen in your big toe, you get nerve pain there. That's because of what happens to the nerve's myelin, a type of insulation that allows the nerve to function more quickly. Myelin is very oxygen dependent. When it lacks sufficient oxygen, it begins to degrade, allowing the nerves to "cross talk." "Cross talk" means that a nerve picks up signals from a nearby nerve and sends a false message to the brain. For example, the breeze from an air conditioner can feel scorching instead of cold. The sensation is not "all in your mind," as many chronic pain patients with strange symptoms are often told. It's a physiological problem of the sympathetic nervous system. But it's far more serious than a mere sensation. Lack of oxygen can lead to a host of ills.

When bone doesn't get the oxygen it needs, it starts to die. That affects any nearby cartilage, which has no circulation of its own and depends on the underlying bone for what it needs. When it is oxygen deprived, cartilage develops subchondral cysts, which are basically dead spots. This degeneration causes pain and inflammation. It's called arthritis.

What major substances contribute to or control pain?

To better grasp the underlying problem of chronic pain and its causes, it helps to understand how certain substances in the body work. Basically, the body produces two harmful substances that contribute to pain and two helpful substances to control pain. Genes determine how much of each substance your body produces. About 25% of the population gets just the right balance, 50% have some imbalance, and the other 25% got the short straw.

Without getting technical, let's focus for a moment on the sympathetic nervous system. It controls blood flow throughout your body. It has a junior partner, norepinephrine, which controls that blood flow for about 20 seconds when you're stressed. He was a handy fellow to have on our side when we lived in caves. His job is to reroute blood from the little muscles, nerves, bones, skin, and gut, and send it to the large muscles so you can fight or run when scared or threatened. We call this the fight or flight response. It was a life-saving reaction in the days when cougars pounced out of trees and instantaneous muscle power was all that could save us.

Today, however, civilization requires that we keep our cool and talk out our differences rather than bashing someone over the head with a club to vent our frustration. Unfortunately, the sympathetic nervous system's junior partner never got that message. That uncomfortable feeling that sweeps through you when you're mad or scared is the junior partner faithfully re-routing your blood flow to the big muscles and cutting off normal circulation to the nerves. You cut off circulation for an extended period of time, and you develop conditions like neuropathies and arthritis. So norepinephrine is one of the bad guys when it comes to chronic pain. The other bad guy is Substance P, the chemical transmitter of pain. People at risk of chronic pain produce too much of this substance. This bad guy lurks in the background waiting for the opportunity to overreact to an injury or some other trigger and play havoc with your sympathetic nervous system.

For our purposes, both of the good guys travel incognito, using only multiple initials to identify themselves. CGRP (calcitonin gene-related peptide) is the major enhancer of circulation to the nerves. To help you remember this guy, think of the letter "C' in his name as standing for "Circulation." The other good guy, VIP (vasoactive intestinal polypeptide), opens the circulation to the gut, which has the ability to distribute helpful substances to all parts of the body. The

> Peptide: a molecule consisting of two or more amino acids.
> Polypeptide: a long chain of peptide molecules.

substances with multiple initials, the good guys, focus on getting blood and its supply of nerve-enhancing oxygen to the nerves.

What happens when your body produces the wrong balance of the pain-controlling substances?

People likely to develop chronic pain produce too much of the bad guys and not enough of the good guys. As a result, these individuals live in a state of heightened reactions to stress. That makes them a potential train wreck of chronic pain just waiting to happen. A chronic stress response means prolonged oxygen deprivation of the nerves. This deprivation eats away at the myelin on the nerves. This loss of myelin leads to "cross talk" between the nerves. Nerves engaging in cross talk indicate a sympathetic nervous system out of whack. And here's the kicker. When the sympathetic nervous system is out of whack, a slight injury, an infection, a bee sting, even a needle prick can push the individual over the edge and into RSD.

Perhaps you can understand now why I attack all areas of pain, large and small, intense or mild, when I treat my patients.

> *"At first I felt silly marking the minor areas of pain on my pain grid. Only after I understood more how the whole process worked did I realize that no hurting was too insignificant to treat. Pain was pain, and Dr. Rhodes needed to treat every bit of it."* *Patti.*

People who come to me have a sympathetic nervous system out of whack. It needs fine tuning all over, not just in the area of perceived pain. I need to put the sympathetic nervous system's junior partner on a short leash, whip Substance P into submission, and call out the two incognito good guys, CGRP and VIP. All of that is done with my treatment modalities. In spite of how it might sound, my methodology is usually painless. I don't like to inflict pain on people already in pain.

However, some patients arrive at my clinic in such deteriorated condition that the diseased area is too sensitive for the patient to tolerate any touch at all. So I cannot place electrodes on them at first. In that case I use an alternative device, a magnetron, which doesn't make physical contact with the skin. If its electromagnetic field also triggers pain repeatedly, I do have a last resort. That is to physically wrap the affected area. That can be painful. But wrapping desensitizes the skin so that the patient can tolerate the electrodes, which then can do their work of normalizing the nerves.

I always stress to my patients the importance of a positive attitude. The body is highly sensitive to negative thoughts. You can understand the mind/body connection easily if you re-call my reference to cougars jumping out of trees to attack early humans. Before claw pierced flesh, the mere sight of the ferocious cat set off an instantaneous surge of norepinephrine in the cave dweller. In other words, the stress response was triggered by a visual cue. It can also be set off by negative thoughts. Therefore, I tell my patients to believe they can recover and to focus on their successes, no matter how slight at first, to keep the bad guys at bay. Everything my pa-tients can do to relieve stress will add to their recovery. With both of us working together, we can look forward to a successful outcome.

HIGHLIGHTS FROM CHAPTER 3

1.   I successfully treat chronic pain caused by lack of oxygen to the nerves.
2.   Successful treatment of chronic pain requires eliminating pain all over the body.
3.   The body produces both harmful substances that contribute to pain and helpful sub-stances that control pain.
4.   People likely to develop chronic pain produce too much of the harmful substances and not enough of the helpful substances.
5.   My treatments are typically painless.
6.   A positive attitude helps the healing process.

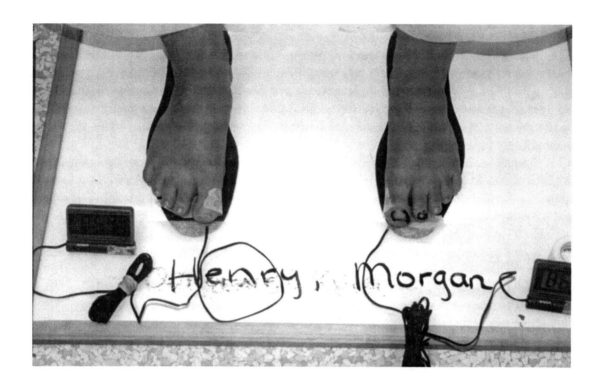

CHAPTER FOUR

NOT KNOWING WHERE YOU'RE GOING UNTIL YOU GET THERE

What I've heard from the skeptics.

When people in pain who have tried every other treatment with no relief hear about me, they are naturally skeptical. They ask questions like, "Who is this guy in Corpus Christi, Texas, who's supposed to be such a hot shot with his pain banishment? Shouldn't I have heard of him? Why doesn't he practice in at least some place like New York City or Los Angeles? What do you mean his treatment is painless? Are you nuts? Every treatment I've had hurt like you-know-what. And all he does is hook you up to some machine he designed, and you get better? Give me a break."

"Our doctor told us not to take our daughter to Dr. Rhodes. We were frantic. No one could help her. So we ignored the advice and went anyway. We are so grateful we did. Dr. Rhodes saved her." Patient's mother.

The first heart transplant took place in South Africa. Who had ever heard of Dr. Christiaan Barnard before he made headlines with his revolutionary approach to treating patients on the brink of death from heart disease?

Marie and Pierre Curie worked alone to discover radium and to experiment with its uses. We wash our hands to get rid of germs due to the findings of Sir Joseph Lister, who startled the world in the 1800's by performing so many operations free of infections. Without Louis Pasteur, we'd risk our health with every glass of milk we drink.

These types of individuals were not thirty-day wonders who one day pulled a revolutionary approach out of a magician's top hat along with the rabbit. Instead, like me, they began with a germ of an idea (pardon the pun), took a shot in the dark that they were on to something, and spent countless years and great effort to hone their research and prove their theory, all for the betterment of humankind. Like most researchers, they often didn't know where they were going until they got there.

To answer the skeptics, I live in South Texas because everybody has to live somewhere, and I happen to live here. I designed my treatment system because of a patient's need and my determination to help her. I had no idea where I was going with my research until I got there. And it's still evolving. I learn new things all the time.

Nuggets of information that led to a surprising conclusion.

Some of the new things I've learned I gleaned from observation of my patients. Others resulted from research of the medical literature. In addition, I have learned a great deal from my clinical studies.

I have observed that the majority of my patients are women. I don't think that's because men are more stoic and less likely to seek help for pain. And it has nothing to do with the outdated concept that women tend to get hysterical. Instead, it is a result of women's physiology.

Remember, nerve pain is caused by a lack of oxygen. Women's bodies do not transmit oxygen from the lungs to the rest of the body as well as men's do because, in general, they have lower blood pressures and lower hemoglobin. Men typically have more muscle than women, which results in more of a substance called myoglobin throughout their body. Myoglobin holds oxygen, so men have more oxygen available to keep their nerves in shape.

I have also observed that, as I treated patients for the pain of RSD, other conditions improved as well. My patients with high blood pressure began getting lower readings. I learned from medical journals that if you create enough CGRP, one of the good guys I have already introduced you to, your blood pressure returns to normal.

Those with asthma and allergies reported a reduction in symptoms. Additional research into the medical literature revealed that people with asthma don't have enough VIP-producing neurons. Pulmonologists treating asthma say if they only had a drug that would release VIP, they could stop asthma. Maybe they should visit with me. Remember, VIP is the other good guy that my protocols prompt the body to produce.

Neurons are nerve cells that send and receive electrical signals over long distances within the body.

More and more, I discovered that treating patients for pain with my approach cleared up a multitude of their other complaints.

I put my observations of these patients together with snippets of information from my research in the medical literature. A surprising conclusion immerged. Many seemingly disparate ailments were actually caused by the same underlying malfunction of the body. And I was treating that basic malfunction with my methods. Migraine headaches, TMJ (a disease of the jaw joint), acid reflux, irritable bowel syndrome, sciatic pain, carpel tunnel syndrome, fibromyalgia, etc.— when I would get one of these conditions to start disappearing in my patients, everything else would follow. No other doctor could do that.

The new perspective on connections between different diseases.

So what's wrong with this picture? What's wrong with it is that medicine has become super specialized. That results in researchers not knowing what other researchers are doing. This disconnect is based on the tremendous amount of information available today. All that information makes it a full time job for medical personnel to stay up to date in their field. They know a great deal about their area but not so much about other areas.

I just happen to be sitting in the middle of all these fields of knowledge and know a little bit about each one. So I have a broader perspective than specialists in particular diseases. It's as if they're separate little villages at the foot of a hill. I'm sitting on the hill, and I can see some of what's going on in each one. Thus, I see connections between the villages that they have not yet recognized. But they're beginning to.

A case in point appeared in the October 12, 2003, issue of *Parade Magazine*, which reported that the medical community recognizes a common, underlying cause for a variety of ailments. In this article, rheumatologist Dr. John Varga, at the University of Illinois in Chicago, explained that doctors in his field realize that the eighty autoimmune disorders are not separate diseases but are all related. These conditions include rheumatoid arthritis, lupus, inflammatory bowel disease, and multiple sclerosis. There are too many others to name.

Another article in a 2006 issue of *Parade Magazine* discussed the use of one specific treatment, acupuncture, to treat a variety of ailments, among them migraines, asthma, menstrual cramps, addiction, and tennis elbow, all of which are related. Now, if they could just figure out the basic cause of this family of ailments as I have.

The point is that new findings in traditional medicine back up what I had already observed in my own practice. Many different types of symptoms in the body stem from the same underlying malfunction. If the body manifests the malfunction as a particular type of chronic pain, it is called RSD. If it crops up in the joints, it's labeled arthritis. If it attacks the lungs, it's diagnosed as asthma. If it sends your blood pressure skyrocketing, it's treated as high blood pressure. The common problem in all these disorders is lack of circulation.

Patients who believe these ailments are separate diseases usually seek a specialist for their diagnosed condition. Treatment typically attacks the symptoms of that one disorder. However, patients who recognize that a host of ailments is caused by the same malfunction will seek a treatment not just for the symptoms, but also for the underlying problem. That's where I come in.

The factor that makes my treatment unique.

As I developed my machine, I used research to reconfigure existing technologies into a new pattern so that I could attack the basic cause of my patients' maladies, which is lack of circulation. I chose frequencies and pulse durations unlike those in any other machine. In addition, instead of targeting the localized area of pain as is done with most electrical stimulation devices, my machine treats the sympathetic nervous system by stimulating the long nerves from one side of the body to other side. That happened because fate must have stepped in.

Let me elaborate by repeating something I previously explained. You may recall that as a podiatrist, I was limited to treating just the ankle and below. Because of that restriction, I had to find a creative way to make that long electrical run through the nerves. I knew that would enhance my treatments. As I have already said, I struggled with how to do that. When inspiration struck and I realized I could send the electricity from one foot to the other, I solved my problem and in the process developed a unique approach. And the enhanced results have been more than I expected

The point is that had I been a doctor licensed to practice on all parts of the body, I might not have opted to make the run all the way to the other side of the body. Yet, that is one of the basic modalities that makes my treatments so successful. In comparison to the TENS, for example, the stimulation from my machine is like the difference between a BB gun and a bazooka. If I have a charging rhinoceros coming at me, personally I'll reach for the bazooka.

> TENS Unit: A medical device that uses electrical stimulation to camouflage the sensation of pain. The electrodes are typically placed near the pain site.

As I further refined what I was doing, I got better and better results. I constantly thought of new pad placements on the body for the electrodes, always aiming for the optimum configuration to get the fastest and best results. I continue that endeavor to this day. Where this will ultimately take me, I don't know. I just know I'll keep going.

What I devised for treatments outside my clinic.

However, in one area of my work, I did know where I wanted to go. In the early days of developing my treatment system, patients had to come straight to me for help. I was the only game in town, or should I say in the world. I treated people who made the trip to Corpus Christi from all over the United States and from as far away as Europe and Australia. They were in so much pain, they would have gone anywhere for relief.

The problem was that in spite of all the patients who left my clinic pain free and stayed that way, some who left pain free lapsed back into RSD. That's due to the nature of the disease. It typically takes six month of continuous treatment to clear up all the underlying malfunctions of the body. In addition, some people are prone to relapses. Continuous or intermittent additional treatment can restore them to health once again, but that meant a return to a tiny spot on the world map, a spot deep in South Texas.

My answer to this problem led me to design a machine for home use. It was smaller and easier to operate than the clinical unit. Patients could buy one, take it home with them, and continue treatment. By the way, since my machine was approved by the FDA as a prescription medical device, patients require a prescription to buy one.

Another idea to provide my treatments to more people involved training other doctors and therapists, who could always call on me for help with difficult cases. Below is a letter from a doctor who wrote to the Kaiser Permanente Medical Group about a patient of his that I had treated. Notice his surprise at the patient's recovery and his interest in learning about my treatments.

February 21, 1999
Dr. Poppert
Kaiser Permanente Medical Group, Outside Referrals
320 Lennon Lane
Walnut Creek, CA 94598

RE: KYLE

DIAGNOSIS: Neuropathic pain/RSD, right ankle.

Dear Dr. Poppert:

By way of summary, I saw Kyle in consultation on 10/25/98. The patient was self-referred after his mother talked to another patient of mine. At that time, I put forth my usual treatment plan to manage this serious neurological problem, and with your kind approval, I started to treat the patient with various pain-relieving procedures as well as medications. With your kind approval, we were also able to obtain physical therapy through the offices of Physical Therapy Specialties. The patient's short course in my practice was characterized by periods of improvement followed by periods of relapse and development of new symptoms like dizziness and myoclonic jerks.

> Myoclonic jerks: involuntary, shock-like contractions or spasms of a muscle or muscle group.

By December, a representative of Physical Therapy Specialties discussed with the patient and his family possible treatment with a podiatrist in Corpus Christi, Texas, that she has visited personally. I looked into the issues as best I could and I discussed this with the patient and his family in detail. At that time, I had very little knowledge of the treatment modalities that the doctor would apply and I was somewhat skeptical based on the claims that I have heard, since I felt that it would be unreasonable for me to prescribe this treatment for a patient of the Kaiser System without having any further information. Nonetheless, the patient's family decided to go to Texas to get this treatment out of great concern for their son. My office stayed in touch with the family and with his physical therapist over the six weeks.

A remarkable story evolved. The patient started feeling better after the first treatment and continued to feel better and apparently had some minor relapse requiring him to stay six weeks instead of four.

He arrives today in my office with his parents and it was extremely remarkable what has transpired.

CLINICAL FINDINGS: Except for continuing atrophy of his right calf, which has also improved, clinical findings were almost back to normal. The temperature of his foot was warm. He had full range of motion and he showed no allodynia. He has been able to go to school and to walk on this leg without any detectable limp. The patient is still weak, but this can easily be resolved by physical therapy, which I feel he should continue at least for another couple of months. The patient does not require any further medications or procedures at this time through my office, but I feel it would be on the side of caution to follow up with him a few more times. I have to say, that in my years of treating RSD and knowing how difficult it is to restore function in these patients, I have yet to see such a sudden, remarkable and complete resolution of symptoms. As a matter of fact, I will be contacting the doctor to look into his methods and possibly visit him in Corpus Christi, Texas.

> Allodynia: pain in response to something that should not cause pain.

If you may wonder why I am writing you this letter today, I think it would be the right thing to do for Kaiser Permanente to reimburse the parents for the out-of-pocket expense that they are looking at. I have to remind you that if the patient had continued treating through more conventional treatments like pain-relieving procedures, medications, etcetera, the ultimate bill probably would have exceeded the family's cost easily. I am delighted for the patient and his parents and I feel humbled in how little we know about RSD, and I am excited about the possibilities that this new treatment may offer.

I will be very happy to have dialogue with you directly, if you require any further information.

Mannie Joel, M.D., M.B., ChB., FRCP. ©
Diplomat – American Board of Anesthesiology
Diplomat – American Board of Pain Medicine
ABA – Certificate of Added Qualifications in Pain Management
Pleasanton, CA

What was my solution for limitations with treatments given outside my clinic?

For a while, I thought that getting my treatment system into the hands of therapists would go a long way toward solving the problem of access. Along with the machine came a set of basic protocols. Protocols are instructions for placement of the electrodes on the body, length of time to run the machine, and frequency settings on the unit. In other words, protocols provide information which therapists need for treatment in the clinic and which patients can use at home.

For more ordinary types of pain, therapists could use the basic protocols with success. But out-of-the-mainstream, stubborn cases and people on medication needed to be referred to me. Some therapists followed through with such referrals. Others did not.

For those patients sent to me, I followed the same procedure I always used with people who didn't respond to established protocols. I dreamed up unique pad placements that only I knew how to design. When I say "dreamed up," that's exactly what I mean. I thought about their symptoms, asked them questions to understand subtle differences in their situation from other patients, and determined, often through trial and error, new electrode placements and machine settings required to solve their particular problem.

Patients on pain medication also require a hands-on approach. Only when patients wean themselves from their pain drugs will they glean optimum benefit from my methodology. That's because medication plays havoc with normal nerve function.

I refused to let these limitations stand in the way of making my treatment available to a much larger population than the numbers of people I could personally treat. So I took out the old brain, dusted it off, and told it to get busy with the answer to yet another problem.

It obliged. Ah, ha! The Internet. Instead of having every patient come to me, I could go to them, virtually speaking. The solution to this particular dilemma lay, first, in developing protocols for every need I could imagine and overcoming the trial and error method of selecting the best protocol for a particular patient. A daunting task, at best. But I've never been smart enough to let that stop me.

The process of selecting the exact protocol for a patient had been less than perfect. That's because of the nature of the nervous system. It's akin to driving from your house to the mall. There's the direct route, which sometimes takes longer because of traffic. You can take the less traveled back route, but the bumpy road drives you crazy. Or you can combine several trips into one and make numerous stops along the way as you traverse a circuitous route to your destination. Just like the trip to the mall, there are many paths through the nervous system. What works best for one person in terms of protocols may not work best for someone else.

I needed some way to predetermine how a particular patient would respond to given protocols. I finally worked out a computer program for this. Before treating patients, I now connect the electrodes from them to a computer and run a series of short tests to determine how they respond to various frequencies and pad placements. The results allow me to hone in on the most likely treatment for that individual's body.

So here I was, seeing my own patients, training a few doctors, and getting a handful of referrals from therapists for difficult-to-treat patients. Yet millions of people in pain could benefit from what I was doing. How could I make my methodology and latest developments available over the Internet to people no matter where they live? I spent a lot of time and research and finally devised a solution. Using the latest technology, I am developing long distance pain banishment.

I have a program that will be available in the future online to care givers everywhere. When this is finalized, you can go local doctors, if they have signed on to offer my treatment and are trained by me, and work through them for an evaluation of your condition. Your physician can oversee your treatment via a hook-up with my clinic. Patients with one of my home treatment machines can check in through their own doctor as needed for follow-ups. This system will revolutionize my practice so that everybody who needs my treatment can have access without having to wait in line outside my office door. It's not a done deal yet, but the mechanisms to put this into place are set up and waiting for the right time. The key is the insurance companies. When they recognize the tremendous savings this treatment offers in contrast to other approaches and how it works when other methods fail, that will open the flood gates for doctors to get involved.

Oh, there's one nice thing about it, too. As I said, this time I know where I'm going before I get there.

HIGHLIGHTS FROM CHAPTER 4

1. As I treated patients for chronic pain, many of their other health complaints improved as well.
2. I realized that many seemingly different health problems are actually caused by the same underlying malfunction.
3. My machine attacks the basic cause of chronic pain, lack of circulation.
4. My treatment is unique.
5. In the future, my treatments may be made available for use by local care givers everywhere via the Internet.

"I was in terrible pain for such a long time. It was worse than childbirth. Then I went to Dr. Rhodes. Once again, I could walk and I could sit. The machine zapped my pain away. It was like the most exciting miracle ever."

Sharon

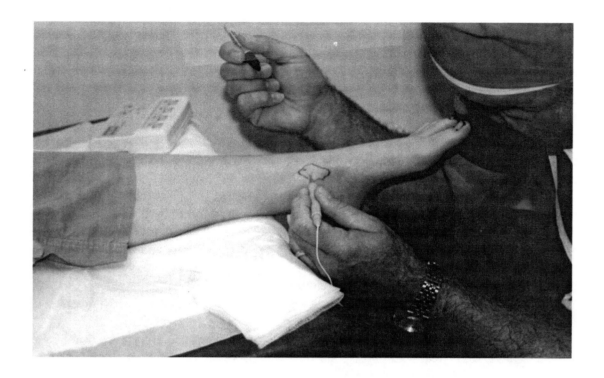

CHAPTER FIVE

THE PROOF IS IN THE PUDDING

Guess what folks back home say about patients who recover from my treatments.

So here I am, successfully treating patients no other doctor has been able to help. Some come to me after surgeries, implants, nerve procedures, heavy-duty pain medications, and a myriad of other interventions--including amputation--have failed or have made them worse. They have spent untold sums of money seeking relief from unrelenting pain. Their life and the lives of their family members have become a shambles. They feel hopeless and helpless. No one knows how to help them. They somehow learn about my clinic, pin their last hopes on me, and make the trip to Corpus Christi, Texas, in a last ditch effort to get their life back.

When they leave my clinic pain free, go home, and resume their daily activities, their friends and colleagues naturally ask what turned their life around. I tell my patients, "When you get home, 19 out of 20 people aren't going to believe my treatment helped you. They may claim it was the placebo effect. For some reason, even though you didn't benefit from the placebo effect before coming to me, they think it has now kicked in big time, and that's why you're pain free.

"Or, they'll say, 'It was *time* for you to get better.' After six years of every treatment under the sun, which made you worse, they're sure something you did before you got to me finally worked. They won't believe that all the fancy, intricate, painful treatments couldn't do what an apparently simple, painless, and non-invasive procedure with a small machine could do."

"One doctor who tried to treat my daughter told me that Dr. Rhodes' machine sounded like voodoo medicine to him. I told that doctor, 'You talk about voodoo medicine. What do you call pumping a thirteen-year-old full of morphine?' No matter what anyone says about Dr. Rhodes, I saw my daughter improve with my own eyes. Nobody can tell me his methods don't work." Mickey.

On the other hand, I've had insurance companies say, "No wonder your patients got better when they never got better with any other treatment. They're down in Corpus Christi sitting in a big chair, and they've got no problems."

I've said, "You've got to be kidding. They're here in Corpus Christi, a beautiful city, but problems don't disappear when you're away from home. They multiply. If you have children, they always seem to get into more mischief when you're not there. Everything that happens around the house is out of your control. You're separated from family and friends. You're not even sleeping in your own bed. You're drinking water which is foreign to you. It's actually a wonder that anybody recovers under those circumstances. Yet, they do."

In addition, insurance companies have said, "Dr. Rhodes, you're so darned radical with this treatment."

I replied, "We are radically constructive with it. If we're not getting results with the way the electrodes and the frequencies on the machine are set, we can change them. It's not like surgery. We didn't cut off somebody's toe and then say, 'You know, I think we'd have gotten better results with the toe on.' Instead, we put the electrode pads in one place, and if we don't think that's going to work well, we just move them to another place until we get it right."

What I had to do to demonstrate my treatments really work.

For a long time, the fact that I knew my patients were recovering was enough for me. When critics claimed I wasn't making a difference, I'd watch a patient walk out the door pain free and say, "I'm making a difference for *that* person." I believe success speaks louder than words. However, I can talk for hours and quote all the peer review journals that show my treatment ought to work the way I say it works. I can refer individuals to patients I have successfully treated. I can bring in doctors to observe my clinic and talk to my patients. But in the final analysis, skeptics want data: number of patients, percentage who improved and how much, and all types of additional statistics. That kind of information requires clinical studies. So I decided the time had come to gather numbers.

First, I wanted a skeptic on board, someone who had no vested interest in positive results. I found this person in Ernesto H. Guido, M. D., a board certified neurologist. In 2001 we set up a study in my clinic. In addition to pain banishment, Dr. Guido decided that we should also check improvement in the transmission and speed of nerve impulses. He didn't think my treatments would make any difference, but he particularly wanted to track F waves anyway. They are the most complicated nerve impulses. They allow us to walk. If there is an F wave in your ankle, it goes up through the nerves in the back, gets redefined, is sent back out through a motor nerve coming back down, and causes a motor contraction. In other words, it triggers a muscle to move.

Since the results of clinical studies are typically cited in percentages, I explained to Dr. Guido how I gauged improvement. Because the medical literature states that the two sides of the body in a healthy person should have a temperature variance of no more than one degree, I first use a specialized machine that tests the temperature of a patient's big toes and the thumbs. I knew from clinical experience that patients in pain came to me initially with a wide variation in those two readings. As they improved, the readings grew closer together.

Second, I conduct painless nerve conduction studies before and after treatment. Healthier nerves conduct better.

Third, I take x-rays of the feet to look for subchondral cysts, a dead give away of malfunction there and in other parts of the body. Remember, RSD is a systemic condition. While the major pain may be confined to a specific part of the body, the entire body is affected.

Fourth, patients fill out a pain grid each day, indicating the location and intensity of their pain. For intensity, we use a scale of 0 to 10, with 0 meaning no pain and 10 the worst pain they can imagine. We ask for their pain level for the top of the foot, the bottom of the foot, hand, arm, elbow, back, knee, etc. Then we ask for the type of pain: burning, numbness, aching. All of these ratings are based on a scale of 1 to 10. We add up the ratings for each type and intensity of pain for an overall score. We compare the score on their first day at my clinic with their score at the end to calculate a percentage of improvement. (See appendix for pain grids.)

I further explained to Dr. Guido that the study would last twenty-eight days. Although most of my patients stay fifteen days in order to start the process of normalizing the sympathetic nervous system, it actually takes at least six months for the body to completely return to normal. Thus, the reason for the home machine. The extra days beyond fifteen in my clinic would allow time for late bloomers to start to blossom before we sent them home. Some patients may experience pain relief the first day while others take longer. That pain relief might last only five minutes at first, perhaps two hours the next day, then longer the day after that, etc. For people on pain killers, the intensity of the pain may lessen slowly before they have any period of total pain relief. No matter what pattern they follow, the goal is to achieve pain relief that lasts twenty-four hours a day. That is best achieved by daily treatments. So we would follow my usual routine of treating patients seven days a week. I have always kept my pain clinic open 365 days a year. That's because pain doesn't take a vacation, and neither do I.

I also explained to Dr. Guido that in spite of all the electronic pain devices on the market, I had discovered the specific pulse durations and frequencies to normalize the body. In addition, traditional electrical stimulation attacks the problem only near the pain site whereas my methodology uses the peripheral nerves to treat the sympathetic nervous system. Not only that, my treatment is individualized for each patient, depending on the person's specific needs.

Why I was told to reject a patient for the study and how I responded.

In spite of all my explanations, Dr. Guido cast a jaundiced eye in my direction. His skepticism resurfaced when we began to screen patients for the study. We put out word locally to find subjects who had long term, unresolved pain. We wouldn't prove anything if we accepted people whose pain was relatively recent. As we scanned the names and medical conditions of those applying, Dr Guido said about one applicant, "Don't put this patient in your study. She's a long term diabetic with lower back pain. She's in her mid-seventies, uses a walker, can't walk without crying, and drags her right foot. No matter what you do, her condition will worsen. Since you obviously won't be able to help her, she will throw off your results."

I replied, "Look, we're dancing. Whoever comes to the dance, we're dancing. If she gets worse during the study, at least we gave her our best shot. If she gets better, that's great." She not only experienced a reduction in her pain, but by the end of the study she also could pick up her right foot and walk with a smile on her face.

This lady was just one of the nineteen out of twenty patients in the study who reported significant pain relief. They ranged in age from thirty-seven to seventy-five. Most of them suffered from diabetic peripheral neuropathy. Remember, all of them had previously failed to respond to other treatments. At the end of the study, seventeen (eighty-five percent) reported an improvement of forty-five percent or greater, eighty percent reported an overall improvement in their quality of life and said they slept better, and forty percent of the subjects were able to significantly reduce their medications. One patient who had peripheral neuropathy for twenty-five years became pain and symptom free. She continues to run her protocols regularly and stays pain and symptom free.

What we did that had never been reported before.

Dr. Guido found, much to his surprise, that more than half of the people had improvement in their nerve conduction. This has never before been reported in the medical literature, particularly in the F waves. If you have an injury that affects the F waves, they may begin working a few months later. But not seven years later from a chronic illness. By they way, you can read the results of our study in the *American Journal of Pain Management,* January 2002.

A second clinical study in 2001 conducted by other doctors, but using my machine and protocols, involved 197 patients, aged twenty-four to eighty-eight. Almost all of them had suffered from chronic pain for at least two years and had tried conventional pain treatments *without* relief. During this study, one third of the participants achieved total pain relief. An additional 58% experienced mild to significant reduction in pain. In other words, over 90% of patients with chronic pain, who had received no help from other methods, responded to my treatments.

The study followed up on about half the patients. Ten percent required no more treatment to remain pain free when contacted ninety days later. Forty five percent opted for treatment as needed while the other forty five percent chose regular treatments to maintain their level of pain relief.

My next study lasted a year and involved only diabetic patients. Not only did I treat their peripheral neuropathy, but I wanted to determine if normalizing their sympathetic nervous system would relieve other malfunctions as well. Diabetics are subject to heart disease, eye problems, poor circulation, infections, and a host of other ailments. I invited several specialists to participate in testing patients before, during, and after their treatments. As we progressed, we got some astounding results, and I learned a great deal. I expect to use that information in a subsequent book.

In addition, I have treated patients with a wide variety of ailments that often involve pain but, in and of themselves, are not just pain syndromes. As these patients have recovered, I have made video tapes of some of their testimonials and posted a few of those on my website at www.paindefeat.com. This information, along with new avenues that open as I treat a broader spectrum of conditions, will also be incorporated into my next book. In it you will read about the upgraded technology and innovative medicine that now being practiced in my clinic.

HIGHLIGHTS FROM CHAPTER 5

1. Skeptics led me to conduct clinical studies to prove my treatment works.
2. The first study involved twenty patients who had failed to respond to other treatments.
3. At the end of the study, nineteen patients reported significant pain relief.
4. A second study conducted by other doctors using my machine involved 197 patients with chronic pain of at least two years' duration.
5. The 197 patients had tried conventional pain treatment without relief.
6. Ninety percent of these patients responded positively to the treatments.
7. A third study, that lasted a year, involved only diabetic patients, who suffered from peripheral neuropathy and other diabetes related conditions.
8. The results of the third study, which were overwhelmingly positive, will be discussed in a subsequent book.

"Dr. Rhodes is helping people no one else can. Everyone who needs his services should have access to them, either from him or from someone he has trained. Insurance companies, distance, and poverty should not be an obstacle. Before they go elsewhere, patients should have the option of going to Dr. Rhodes first."

Suzanne

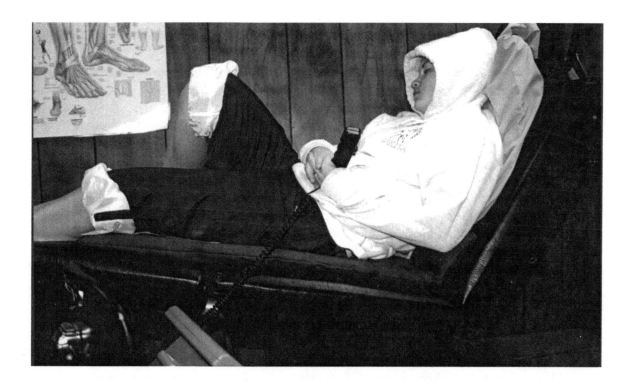

CHAPTER SIX

HOPING TO FAIL AN EXAM

How do I determine if a pain condition can respond to my treatments?

People all over the country contact me, asking if I can help them. Whether they suffer from RSD, the diabetic pain of peripheral neuropathy, after effects of an operation, arthritis, fibromyalgia, etc., I ask them a series of questions about their diagnosis, treatments to date, and current medications. From that I determine if they are a potential patient. If so, I explain that if they decide to come to my clinic, I will perform a series of objective, painless tests. If they fail particular ones, I know their sympathetic nervous system (SNS) is out of whack, exactly the condition my protocols treat.

Tests include painless neurometer studies. For this, electrodes are attached to the toes, one at a time. Electrical stimulation is sent to each toe while a meter registers intensity. The greater the intensity before the patient feels any sensation, the less nerve conduction the patient has. When a patient fails by responding at an abnormally high setting, I have the first indication that this is someone I can successfully treat.

Next, I have the patient stand on a thermal pad that registers the temperature of the feet to help determine circulation. Another circulation test, the IMEX, registers the blood flow in the lower extremities. Some people with poor circulation register nothing.

I also check the temperature of the two big toes and the pads of the two thumbs. I mentioned before that the temperature variation between the right and left side of the body should be no more than one degree. The greater the temperature difference between the two sides of the body, the more severe the impairment of the SNS.

Then, I x-ray the feet. Remember those subchondral cysts I told you about earlier? When the SNS has gone off the deep end, those cysts appear all over the body. If I find them in the feet, I know they are spread throughout the body, also. A patient who fails these tests is a prime candidate for my clinic. This is probably the first time they hope to fail an examination. That's because not passing means they have come to the right place.

"My symptoms were so weird that I thought I might be suffering from Lyme disease. I read that it comes from a spirochete that, after treatment, hides away in cysts in the body and then breaks out periodically to cause havoc. When I went to Dr. Rhodes, I learned that I did have cysts. However, they came not from Lyme but from RSD. How many people who believe they have long-term Lyme disease actually suffer from RSD triggered by Lyme?" A patient.

What commitment do the patient and possibly other family members need to make?

I can probably help other members of the individual's family who have chronic health problems. Here's why. Keep in mind that, genetically, some individuals are more prone to chronic pain than others. Those people typically come from a family with ailments such as allergies, asthma, arthritis, fibromyalgia, migraines, endometriosis and carpel tunnel syndrome. These conditions are caused by a sympathetic nervous system out of whack. By contrast, you could say that the intensity of RSD-type pain reflects the SNS gone berserk. However, in both cases, the treatment is the same. What varies is the length of time required to normalize the SNS so the person can function free of symptoms. While some people respond in a matter of weeks with a permanent recovery, others can take up to six months, even longer sometimes.

When I say normalizing the SNS can require up to six months, I am talking about daily treatments that gradually reduce the pain and then keep it in check while the body continues its work of healing. During this recovery period, I recommend twice-a-day treatments. That involves my home machine, which allows the patient to continue treatment without having to come to my clinic every day. So, whether it's the patient in pain or family members with other symptoms, a commitment to continued use of the protocols at home is important for full recovery.

What actually happens during my office treatments?

Before I begin treatments, I perform other tests to determine the choice protocols and the frequency best suited to the individual patient. I previously mentioned this procedure as one of the enhancements to my practice. It involves a series of four-minute tests carried out over several days until we finally pinpoint the exact machine settings and pad placements that will give the patient the fastest results.

"I believe I was one of the most difficult patients Dr. Rhodes has treated. I was in severe pain, and my right hand was knotted in a fist I couldn't open. My body was so damaged from morphine I took for pain, and I had been through so many procedures, that I responded very slowly. However, I never gave up. I would go home at times and

then come back, ready to try again. Finally, it happened. Dr. Rhodes developed a new approach that made the difference for me. It was when he did the testing for the best frequencies and pad placements that I really started to improve." Nicole.

First, you rate your pain.

Each day before using the protocols, the patient fills out a pain grid. (See Appendix.) This indicates the worst areas of pain plus all milder pain. It includes a number from one to ten to indicate pain intensity. Remember, I treat every twinge, one area at a time. I start with the worst pain and then chase down all the other, little pains. RSD can be insidious. It can spread, taking up residence in one part of the body and then hiking to another part. I can snuff it out, and it can roar back. Or it may slink away, never to be heard from again. Everybody's different. So each person's treatment must be individualized. And the time required to recover varies greatly.

Then, we make you comfortable.

As for treatments in my clinic, we provide patients with overstuffed recliners so that they sit comfortably while hooked to the machine. I sometimes call my clinic the chain saw factory or the "Z-Zone" because most patients fall asleep during treatment, so they're getting their z-z-z-z's. They nod off because the machine produces VIP. Do you remember my discussion of the good guys and the bad guys? You may recall that VIP is a good guy. One of its functions is to work on the pineal gland in your head to create melatonin, a sleep inducer. Since chronic pain patients are typically sleep deprived, the ability to catnap during protocols is a bonus. Not only do patients feel better, but they heal faster since most healing takes place while we sleep.

You relax during treatments.

Each protocol takes from twenty to forty minutes. Protocols alternate between the lower and upper body. In other words, while you relax in a recliner, a technician hooks you up for treatment by first placing electrodes on specific sites on your feet or legs, ramping up the electrical impulses from the machine until you can feel tingling without pain, and then setting the timer on the machine for twenty or forty minutes, depending on the protocol. When the timer buzzes, the electrodes are moved to the hands or arms, the impulse is reset to a comfortable intensity, the required time is keyed in on the machine, and you relax and can get some more z-z-z-z's for another 20 to 40 minutes, if you care to. The first day in my clinic is usually the longest because of all the testing prior to running the first protocols.

If you take pain medications, we wean you off of them.

Patients who come to me on narcotic-type pain medication must be weaned off those drugs before treatment can be truly successful. In the early days, such people began treatments, gradually decreased their meds, but finally reached a point where they had to suffer the agonies of withdrawal to clear their system completely. That part of the procedure always troubled me. Remember, I offer painless help. I conducted more research, experimented, and finally broke new territory. Now, I have learned how to bring patients down off those narcotics without withdrawal symptoms. However, due to the nerve damage from those meds, their pain recovery is typically longer.

To check your progress, we retest you.

To gauge their progress, I retest all patients periodically during treatment and before I release them to go home. In addition to their own reports of improvement, the tests give me objective evidence of their condition. A funny situation took place several years ago when I was treating two young girls from different parts of the country. The periodic tests of the girl who arrived first and had been treated longer showed marked improvement, in spite of the fact that the girl continued to report a high level of pain. I was puzzled about the discrepancy. Only when she was caught acting normal did she confess. She and the other girl had become such good friends in my clinic that the girl who arrived first for treatment kept reporting pain after it had been eliminated so that her family wouldn't take her home. The tests had been truthful, but she hadn't.

Let me be clear. Many patients leave pain free after 15 days of treatment. Some never need to return or use the machine again. Others find that to retain their improvement, they must continue using the machine at home, at least for six months. Then there are those whose pain goes into remission but crops up again due to a minor accident, an illness, or for no apparent reason. They would be well advised to run the machine regularly, as I do every day.

Guess what health condition I share with my patients.

Yes, I use my machine on a regular basis. After a bout of RSD of my own due to an arm injury, I realized I felt better and remained healthier by following a maintenance schedule I devised for myself after I put my own RSD into remission.

I won't go into my RSD story here. Instead, I'm going to let some of my patients tell you in their own words what happened to them. The people I've treated have ranged from individuals with ordinary chronic pain to patients who have almost died. If you suffer as they have, you may find a story here similar to yours. If so, I trust learning about others who have triumphed over what you are now enduring will give you hope that, yes, a viable treatment for your agony exists.

HIGHLIGHTS FROM CHAPTER 6

1. Before I treat patients, I run tests on them that indicate whether my treatment is likely to help them.
2. Then I run tests that indicate the best protocols and machine settings for each individual.
3. Before treatment, patients fill out a pain grid.
4. Patients sit in overstuffed recliners during treatment.
5. Patients on pain medication must be weaned off their drugs for treatment to be successful.
6. Normalizing the SNS typically takes six months of continuous at-home use of the machine.
7. Some patients will need to continue treatments on a long-term basis beyond six months to stay pain free.

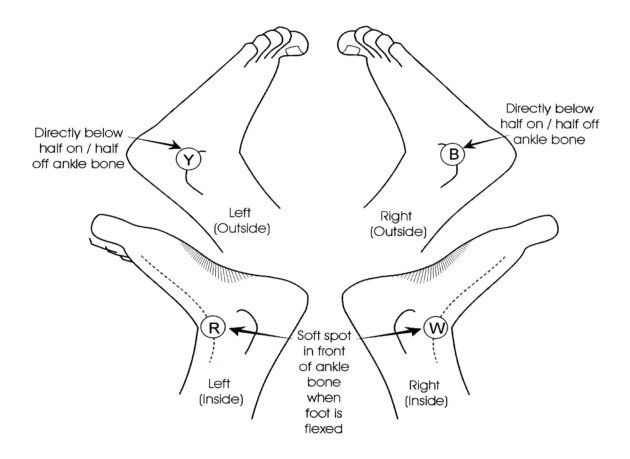

Directly below half on / half off ankle bone — **Y**

Directly below half on / half off ankle bone — **B**

Left (Outside)

Right (Outside)

R ← Soft spot in front of ankle bone when foot is flexed → **W**

Left (Inside)

Right (Inside)

CHAPTER SEVEN

LOOKING BACKWARD AND FORWARD AT THE SAME TIME

Just how successful are my treatments?

I am often asked just how successful my treatments are. I can't speak for therapists who have used my approach in other settings. Most of them don't have the equipment to run the preliminary tests that I do, nor can they determine the best protocols and machine settings for the individual patient. However, as I pointed out earlier, I have set up a system to overcome that problem through primary care physicians and therapists. When they sign on to offer treatments via an Internet hookup with my clinic, I'll be able to provide services through them that they have not been able to offer.

As for my clinic, quantifying a success rate depends on what you mean by success. Most patients respond to my treatments. By most, I would say over ninety percent. By respond, I mean that over 90 percent improve. They feel better, they experience less pain, and most eventually achieve pain free status, which is always my goal. What I cannot report is how many patients continue to use the therapy after they leave my clinic. I advise long term use for roughly an hour-a-day of a maintenance protocol at home. In addition, those who stay in contact with my office and have flare ups can fax me pain grids if problems arise. If they use the protocols I fax back, most can expect to regain their pain free status. Some patients have done well for years and then reinjured themselves and relapsed. Because I continue to refine what I do, they usually return for upgraded treatments. They can look forward again to restored health.

The key is to recognize that the body is like a big battery. It needs recharging. Wear and tear, stress, the daily demands of living wear down systems in the body, making it vulnerable to aches and pains. Injuries, illnesses, and other traumas can short circuit a body under such stress and turn aches and pains into chronic, intractable pain. And that's where I come in. My therapy works to correct the short circuit when the SNS blows a fuse.

Why should a patient come to me for treatment first rather than last?

If you quantify success by how well I help patients no other doctor as been able to help, my success rate shoots off the charts. Keep in mind, most of my patients come to me *after* many failed, traditional treatments. Those patients have been 100% failures with their previous therapies. In my clinic, 90% of them respond positively. However, such patients will take longer to heal. If they had known to come to me first, instead of last, I could have helped them before their nerves were damaged from narcotics, their bodies were sliced open and sewn up after implants, or they gave up limbs to amputation in a desperate attempt to relieve their suffering.

What do patients need to know about insurance coverage for my treatments?

Patients also want to know if insurance will cover my treatments. Most companies will. We gladly check the coverage of prospective patients so they will know what to expect in that regard. In the early years, many companies considered what I was doing experimental, although electrical stimulation for a variety of conditions was a recognized, safe therapy. Even though my machine was approved by the FDA for pain control, I had long conversations with insurance companies, who paid enormous sums for operations and other invasive procedures that can't help anyone with RSD-type pain since any trauma to the body only worsens RSD and its related ills. Yet in the past, insurance companies balked at paying for a much less expensive form of therapy in my clinic. However, today, the picture has improved. Patients may have to spend some money out of pocket, but the major cost usually no longer falls on their shoulders.

"The ability of Dr. Rhodes to successfully treat RSDS is of great importance to me because I have a sister, Cathy, who has suffered with RSDS for over eighteen years. She has undergone eleven surgeries and over one hundred and fifty blocks. None of these traditional treatments helped Cathy. In fact, in almost every case, these treatments only enhanced the disease. The expense for this failed care has been astronomical. The insertion of a morphine pump cost well over fifty thousand dollars. This alone makes Dr. Rhodes' successful treatment very important. He puts an end to the exorbitant medical expenses, and the patient is no longer forced to endure unnecessary and harmful operations, physical therapy, or blocks and medications." Barbara.

What are the side effects of electromagnetic stimulation of the sympathetic nervous system?

I am often asked about side effects of my treatments. Over the many decades that various forms of electrical stimulation have been used, the medical literature has reported few, if any, negative effects. In my own practice, I have found that occasionally a few patients experience some slight nausea. But that is easily treated with anti-nausea protocols. It has been reported in other offices that some patients may develop a temporary, irregular heartbeat that returns to normal after a few more sessions with the machine. Patients who ramp up the intensity of the stimulation too high can experience a transitory buzzing of the nerves and ringing in the ears. That after-effect is self-limiting. As far as serious side effects, I know of none.

What do I foresee for the future in regard to my treatments?

Some people ask me when I'm going to reach the pinnacle of refinements with my treatments. I can only say, looking backward and forward at the same time, that I envision a continuing compendium of enhancements from my first patient to whoever will be my last. After all, researchers in cancer, heart disease, immunology, and other fields never believe they have "arrived." They continue to look for new and better methods, drugs, and treatments.

I have already devised protocols to treat multiple areas of the body at the same time. I have plans for a day when, instead of using separate electrodes, the patient will put on something like gloves and socks with imbedded electrodes, making protocols easier to use. The final step in this regard would be a wireless system. That is not beyond the realm of possibility. In fact, it's a basic idea already attributed to someone else. John Sutherland, dean of the Boston University School of Medicine, is reported to have described in 1912 a feature of the house of the future. He said it would be "equipped with electrical apparatus which will, without the inmates knowing it, keep them constantly charged with electricity, thereby warding off many of the ills and aches that flesh has hitherto been heir to."

I also have plans to target more specifically the exact spot where the patient hurts and administer a protocol that works almost instantly. Beyond that, I look forward to the time when we can genetically determine those people most likely to develop chronic pain. We can then offer preventive intervention instead of waiting until an individual's SNS falls off the deep end. Where all these upgrades will take me, I can only imagine. But if I told you the totality of what I see in the future, I'm sure you'd be skeptical. So instead of spelling out what I conceive is possible and achievable, I'm going to stop here with what has already been accomplished.

After I have more solid evidence on the scope of what my treatment system is capable of doing in areas other than pain banishment, I'll be back with more information and patient stories. Until then, I can report briefly the results of my latest study involving diabetic Type 2 patients. This study was presented at the National Clinical Meeting of the Diabetes Technology Society in Atlanta, Georgia, during November 2006, and was published in their peer reviewed journal.

Utilizing both objective and subjective measurements taken throughout the course of the study, it was demonstrated that my therapy is effective in retarding the progression of, and in some cases reversing certain effects of, diabetes throughout the body. Among the areas of improvement were diabetic osteoporosis, diabetic nephropathy, diabetic neuropathy, hypertension, and hyperglycemia. My goal is to conduct a larger diabetes study in the near future to explore further the full potential of sympathetic therapy in reversing this disease.

Now, let me introduce you to a few of the multitude of "hopeless" individuals who have crossed my clinic threshold in terrible pain and have had their life restored. Some of them have completed treatment while others are in the midst of getting well. They and their families will tell you their stories in their own words.

HIGHLIGHTS FROM CHAPTER 7

1. Over ninety percent of my patients improve, with many becoming pain free, which is always my goal.
2. Patients who relapse can usually be retreated with success.
3. Although most of my patients come to me as a last resort after standard treatments for pain have failed, most recover.
4. The majority of insurance companies cover my treatments.
5. I know of no serious side effects from my treatments.
6. I anticipate future expansion of the use of sympathetic therapy.
7. Some of my patients and their families will tell their story in their own words.

PART TWO—MIRACLE REMISSIONS

Below are stories from a few of my patients, told in their own words.

Patricia Boeckman

Corpus Christi, Texas

I woke up in the middle of the night with my entire body, face, cheeks, and scalp buzzing like a bee hive gone mad. My nerves burned like fire. My ears were ringing so loudly I was almost deaf to everything else. What was happening to me? I felt certain I'd wake up the next morning totally paralyzed.

The year was 1993. Eight days after a flu shot, I began to feel sick and experienced strange sensations in my feet. I could have sworn they were blistered on the bottom. Then vibrations, coupled with what can only be described as something akin to bolts of electricity, began to spread up my legs. I developed fasciculations, which are twitches in the muscles.

My mind became foggy, my memory was shot, and I felt wretched most of the time. Every nerve in my body constantly burned and stung. My ears rang continuously. I lived with a perception of extreme weakness, but I was fully able to climb stairs as usual. However, I had no energy. I had bouts of feeling desperately ill, so sick that many times I almost called an ambulance to take me to the hospital. Something was severely wrong, something that I thought required tubes leaking medicine of some kind into my veins. But after a while, that sensation would pass, and I would feel only miserable, not desperate, so I never made any 911 calls.

Eventually, I woke up on two separate nights a few days apart from bizarre sensations I had never before experienced. Every nerve in my body was humming and vibrating like a piano string which had been struck violently and refused to settle down. My nerves felt on fire. This feeling consumed my entire body, including my face, my tongue, my scalp, and my ears, which screamed with a high pitched buzzing. I was sure it would drive me crazy. My whole nervous system felt under assault by some unseen monster. The two nights were the same, yet somehow different. Both times I was actually shocked when I awoke the next morning able to move and get out of bed.

Doctors gave me various tests, none of which pointed to a specific diagnosis. I felt miserable. Still, I could function on some level, so I plodded on with my life, which became a blur of depression, great sadness for the basically healthy individual I had once been, and bewilderment at what ailment I could possibly have. Sure, I had a few minor chronic conditions like many people, but nothing like the all-encompassing shroud of never-ending nerve pain that had kidnapped my life and held me hostage.

Then in 1999 a doctor put me on neurontin, and the symptoms receded. I eventually felt well enough to try to wean myself off the medication, but every attempt plunged me back into the nightmare existence I had taken the medicine to alleviate. So I finally realized I would have to take it the rest of my life. It did not cure me. But it did keep me comfortable.

Fortunately, in 2001 I heard about a local doctor who had designed a machine to banish pain. Both my husband and I were suffering from severe shoulder pain at the time. I was on summer break from teaching and wondered how I could possibly do my job with severe hurting that refused to abate. My husband had received three months of conventional therapy to no avail and had already been given a discouraging prognosis--that no treatment would alleviate his pain, so he would have to live with it for the rest of his life. With nothing to lose, we decided to give the local doctor a try.

After two weeks of treatment, both my husband and I walked out of Dr. Rhodes' clinic pain free. To this day, neither of us has been troubled with a recurrence.

But I walked away with more than a pain-free shoulder. In the two weeks I sat in Dr. Rhodes' clinic hooked up to his machine, I talked to other patients whose stories fascinated me. Over and over I heard them comment that someone should write a book about this amazing doctor. As a writer with an extensive publishing background, I decided that someone should be me.

I was so intrigued that I hung around Dr. Rhodes' office off and on and began to interview his patients. Gradually, I grasped something of the scope of what this Miracle Man was doing as I watched patients wracked with pain enter his clinic and leave restored to health or on their way to recovery and singing his praises.

Finally, I realized that his treatments resolved a wide variety of ailments, all related, but each masquerading as a separate disease. When he talked about how his extensive research had led him to the modalities that he used to banish types of chronic pain that almost nobody understood, I was struck by his brilliance.

Then I asked him if he could resolve the nerve condition that I kept in check with neurontin. He said yes. As he treated me, I gradually got off the medication, and I haven't taken a dose of it since 2002.

For a number of years, I had also lived with flare ups of an arthritic condition that bounced around to several sites on my body, and I had intermittent, exquisitely painful wrists and chronic neck discomfort. I also had developed an overactive bladder, for which I was told by my urologist that I would "be on" medication, which meant indefinitely. I had a painful foot disorder called Morton's Neuroma, which had been operated on years earlier, to no avail. Just trying on a pair of high heels was so intensely painful that I had worn nothing but flats for twenty years.

Dr. Rhodes designed specific protocols for me to knock out the pains and the bladder trouble. The treatments worked, tuned up my body like an old car made to purr again, and made me feel years younger. In addition, I tossed away the bladder pills, and for the first time in two decades, I could put on a pair of high heels and walk off without even a twinge in my feet.

I have turned out to be the type of patient who needs to keep Dr. Rhodes' machine on hand to recharge my batteries when they begin to sputter out, but I have long periods when I have barely an ache of any kind and do not need to "zap," as I call it.

I have learned to be kind to my body to help maintain my recovery. For example, I do not ingest caffeine and try to avoid highly acidic foods to keep mild ear ringing and tingling feet at bay. I try to get enough sleep. I take vitamins. I eat a well-balanced diet.

I represent patients who have had more tolerable levels of pain than some of those you will read about here. Their dramatic stories take you through torturous situations no human being should have to endure. But they also offer hope that individuals suffering from intractable agony can rise again from their wheel chairs and beds of suffering and participate once again in life.

The stories that follow come from patients and their families themselves. Not content to rely totally on stories from only the most recent of Dr. Rhodes' patients, I was able to contact many of his earliest clients to question them about their current status. I wanted readers to know whether results could be long lasting. I was quite impressed with how well these patients were doing. And their improvement involved more than just pain banishment. For example, one fellow whose story is not in this book was treated a few years ago by Dr. Rhodes for diabetic neuropathy. During the course of his treatments, he discovered a marvelous improvement he hadn't anticipated. His kidney function, which had deteriorated to 50% of normal due to diabetes, returned to 100%. Several years after he stopped using the machine, his kidney function remained at 100%. His regular doctors were amazed and couldn't understand how such a change was possible. But he knew.

I spoke with most of Dr. Rhodes' patients in person, others I phoned, and a few sent me their stories via email. Some preferred that I use only an initial or a first name. One person specifically asked to be identified with her full name, city, and state.

You will find these true stories compelling. Each one offers a new bit of insight or some tidbit you won't find anywhere else in this book. I hope what you read here will help you or someone you love.

Footnote:

The original intent of this book was to help people interested in Dr. Rhodes' treatments to understand what his treatments involve, how he got into pain banishment, and what to expect if they came to Corpus Christi to get help from him. Also, it was to give enthusiastic patients something concrete to hand to other sufferers to encourage them that they could overcome their pain, even when nothing else had worked. This book has served that purpose many times over.

However, after getting feedback for some time on the first version of PAIN BANISH-MENT, I realized that another goal was equally important. This book could help serve as a vehicle to bring Dr. Rhodes the kind of recognition he needs to generate funds for large-scale studies to prove to the medical community what his treatments can do. When powerful people in the medical field have to sit up and take notice that this one man has developed a technology that is helping patients no one else has been able to successfully treat, that this is a low-cost modality compared to heavy-duty therapies that just make patients worse, and that this approach can be learned and used all across the country and the world, then health care costs will plummet. The number of people suffering from a host of treatable maladies that dumbfound traditional medicine will also plummet. And the world will be a better place for all.

If you have the means to help make this happen, I urge you to act. Spread the word about Dr. Rhodes. Write your legislators and ask for funding for large clinical trials. Contact foundations that give grants. Talk to your insurance company about this cost-saving treatment. Send a copy of this book to someone you think may be in a position to help. By assisting in this endeavor, you could be helping yourself. That's because even if you are in perfect health today, you could need this treatment tomorrow. None of us knows when or whom intractable pain will strike.

~~~~~

Harley, the Million Dollar Man

Dallas, Texas

June 19, 1994, would eventually become the most expensive day of my life. By the time I turned 60 seven years later, I was looking back at medical bills that topped $1,000,000.

I drove gasoline tankers. My problems all started when I was putting a hose back on a tanker. I stepped on a little bitty rock. I fell with a twisting motion. I used my right arm to brace myself and broke my elbow. I fractured my wrist and damaged my cervical thoracic and lumbar spine. I went first to the doctor and then to the hospital. Because my arm hurt more than my back, they x-rayed my arm but not my spine.

I was treated for my arm injury and pain by an orthopedist for six months. I developed a purple, splotchy right hand. The doctor never picked up on what it was. He thought it was carpel tunnel syndrome. He and a second doctor, who said I had RSD, totally disagreed on the diagnosis. I fell into a nightmare of problems with workman's compensation insurance, which doctors I was allowed to see that the insurance would cover, conflicting advice from various doctors about treatment, being scheduled to see a psychologist to learn "pain management," one doctor canceling another doctor's orders because of insurance limitations, and a nurse case manager firing everybody who treated me and starting me with yet another doctor.

The stress was incredible, and the pain was spreading from my elbow toward my shoulder. Finally, the next doctor, who treated RSD patients, started me on a series of injections for the pain. They helped somewhat.

Then I began to hurt in the lumbar spine area. I received ganglion blocks for the next year. Meanwhile, I developed brain fog and more pain, suffered from both depression and lack of sleep, and learned that my nurse case manager had been removed from my case by the insurance company.

Then I had a battle with the insurance company. It began to deny treatment. Although I had hurt my back in my initial fall, that had been ignored since my arm had originally been the main area of concern. So the insurance company claimed my back was not part of the original injury.

I deteriorated to the point I could no longer walk unaided and needed a wheel chair. The insurance company said no. My daughter provided one for me. A paralegal, she was so overcome with frustration at the way I was treated that she began to focus her practice on the workman's compensation field. Her help through this whole ordeal has been invaluable to me.

The next doctor I was sent to took back x-rays and used very conservative spine manipulation treatments. When an order for a CAT scan of my upper and lower spine was sent to the insurance company, they denied it. The doctor ordered it again, and it was approved. The tests showed a bulged disk in the spine and other spinal damage. When the doctor said I needed surgery, the insurance company once again said no, that it was not part of my injury.

I took my case to the Texas Workman's Compensation Commission. They agreed my back problem was work related. However, it took two years of arguing with the insurance company to get them to admit it. During that time, I went to six or seven hearings. Eventually, the insurance company was fined for non-compliance.

Finally, I had the spinal surgery. After a year of therapy, I was out of the wheel chair.

Then I began to deteriorate. My legs began to give away. I fell and tore the meniscus in my right knee. I had surgery on it twice. I developed RSD after that. My feet were swollen. I was in pain, including chest pain like a heart attack. I was in and out of the emergency room. But I had no diagnosed heart problems. I later learned my symptoms came from pain in sympathetic nerves near my heart.

I was getting worse, not better. So I was referred to a pain specialist in Florida to determine the best medications and dosages to help relieve my pain. I took the highest dosage of neurontin, 4,800mg a day, plus other pain pills. The pain actually leveled out. For a while. Then it roared back and got totally out of control. I was having blinding headaches on top of everything else.

I saw so many doctors and had so many therapies I can't recall them all. I do recall that I had prolotherapy, which was excruciatingly painful, went to a quack who said pumping my arm up and down in a certain way followed by a series of shots in my stomach would take away the pain, and was told I needed a sympathectomy. There seemed to be no end to the recommendations, and they were all different. Didn't anybody have an answer?

Next I tried a doctor in Dallas. He told me I was a good candidate for a morphine pump. I was desperate and ready to try anything. It did help for a while. Then I fell again and tore my meniscus a second time. My feet and legs swelled up like balloons. I was in so much pain I couldn't tolerate wearing support hose to try to lessen the swelling. My whole existence was PAIN and more PAIN. I was put in a compression machine, which did help somewhat. But I couldn't get one through the insurance company to use at home.

Three doctors ordered me a motorized wheel chair. The insurance company denied it. We insisted on a medical review. We won, but a year later, I still don't have the chair.

Through a series of contacts, my daughter learned about Dr. Rhodes. I had been to so many doctors by then, had undergone outlandish and harmful procedures, had been operated on, medicated until I was an unthinking, unresponsive zombie, that I thought this was just another witch doctor. I had had enough of that. But my daughter checked Dr. Rhodes out and urged me to give him a try.

With no hope left, I allowed my wife to take me to Corpus Christi to see Dr. Rhodes. He said he could help me. He also told me it would take time, because I would have to get off the morphine and all narcotic type medication. They work against the machine. In a month I dropped from 16 milligrams of morphine a day to 6 milligrams. My mind became clearer. I could think. Eventually, I had to totally stop the morphine. The detox process was horrible. Sometimes I thought I wasn't going to make it. But I did. With my wife's support, I stayed with it. Also, something about Dr. Rhodes and hearing the success stories of other patients gave me the determination to stick it out. And I knew he was customizing his treatments just for me since the same protocols don't necessarily work for everyone.

In two months, Dr. Rhodes worked a miracle. I went from full body pain so intense I would have gladly died to no pain except for my right knee. For the first time since 1994, I was basically pain free. Home treatments would take care of what was left of the knee pain.

I went home, treated myself regularly, and then returned later to have the morphine pump removed. I wanted to be under Dr. Rhodes' care in case the surgery triggered the RSD again. There were some complications involving the surgery, but Dr. Rhodes took care of them.

Dr. Rhodes' treatment is great. I'm 100 percent sold on it. I can play with my grandchildren again. I can look forward to tomorrow and the day after that. I can smile and laugh, think and plan, and enjoy my time on this earth. It's given me back a quality of life I thought I'd lost forever.

~~~~~~

Marcia

Corpus Christi, Texas

On Friday, November 9, 2001, I went to bed fine and woke up the next morning literally unable to move.

My story begins in Alexandria, Virginia, winter 1953, when I was six years old. Mother says she had no idea anything was wrong until she bathed me that night. My left knee was swollen to twice its normal size. The school said that I had fallen off a snow sled, so mom chalked it up to the usual scrapes and bumps that befall a six-year-old. However, the swelling continued to worsen. The doctors drained the fluid several times, but it would always come right back. Fearing I might have TB of the bone, the doctors scheduled me for exploratory surgery in August, 1953. In that surgery, they performed a synovectomy and diagnosed rheumatoid arthritis. After that my left leg was in a cast or a brace nearly all the time, and I was in and out of hospitals as doctors tried to straighten the knee that fused after the surgery. Other joints quickly became involved: my left ankle, my right knee and right ankle. I began a regimen of cortisone and aspirin. Swelling and pain and the inability to do the physical things my friends could do became my reality. But with a child's faith and my parents' positive thinking, I weathered those early years and made it to puberty without needing the wheelchair that the doctors had predicted would be my future.

With puberty came more inflammation, more pain, and more joint involvement. But the casts and braces were off and I rarely needed crutches. The doctors tried various drug treatments, but I responded best to aspirin.

With the exception of a major flare up during college, my rheumatoid arthritis remained quiet until after the birth of our son in 1969. After that the disease spread to all my joints, even my jaw! I saw doctors and tried different medications. Nothing worked very well. In 1970 I had surgery on my right knee. In a way I was very lucky to have this disease hit so early. I adjusted to chronic pain when I was too young to even remember, and so having pain all the time was natural. I didn't let it dictate what I could or couldn't do. However, as the years passed, the pain reached levels that became more and more difficult to live with. The medications the doctors tried were stronger and stronger.

In 1976, the pain was making my life miserable. I was teaching and on my feet all day. My knees and ankles were a mess. I made an appointment to see Dr. Rhodes. He watched me walk and said he could make orthotics for me that would change the way my muscles, tendons, and ligaments pulled on my knees. What a miracle!! They worked wonderfully!! With the orthotics, the pain receded. Unfortunately, over time, my legs began to adjust to the orthotics. Dr. Rhodes would adjust them, and I would be good to go again. Eventually, however, the orthotics alone were not enough, so in 1980 I started using a tens unit to control the pain. This worked as long as I had it on. When I turned it off, the pain was back.

In 1985, I had my third knee surgery. This time an arthroscopy was used to attempt to control the pain and swelling in my left knee and postpone having a total joint replacement. I was 38 years old. From 1985 until 2001 the disease was never under control. My days started and ended with pain, swelling, and stiffness. Doctors prescribed different pain relievers as they came on the market, but nothing worked very well. During these years I lost more and more motion.

On Friday, November 9, 2001, I went to bed fine and woke up the next morning literally unable to move. Rheumatoid arthritis has a nasty habit of exploding on you suddenly. Nothing on my body worked. My hands were completely numb. I couldn't use my fingers to pick up anything. I couldn't comb my hair. I couldn't dress myself. I couldn't get into or out of a chair without assistance. I couldn't walk. I couldn't do anything. And the pain was incredible. My husband put me in a hot tub for thirty minutes. I started to move. About two hours later I could think.

I tried to see a rheumatologist in town. They were booked solid for six to eight months. That was awful. So I saw a wonderful rheumatologist in San Antonio, and the medication she put me on gave me my life back. I was taking prednisone, methotrexate, and hydrocodone. This mixture worked well for a while. Then I started needing higher doses of everything to keep my body working. In May 2002, I was diagnosed with thyroid cancer, which the doctors felt was caused by the methotrexate. In July I had the right lobe of my thyroid gland removed. Shingles are also a side effect of the medicine, and I had a really bad attack of those. I was suddenly on a very serious downward spiral.

My arthritis symptoms continued to get worse and worse. I had an anaphylactic reaction to the methotrexate and had to stop taking it all at once. In its place, I began taking neurontin. I needed more and more medication to make it through a day. I was taking 7.5/750mg of hydrocodone every 2 hours and 100mg of neurontin every day, and together they were not enough to control the pain. And my liver function tests were coming back abnormal. The pain was out of control and so was my arthritis. I was miserable and I was desperate.

The doctor said the next step was knee replacement surgery. Because I've had this disease since I was six, I have osteoporosis and am not a good candidate for that kind of surgery. I'm an RN. I worked in the OR. Knee and hip replacement surgery I see every day. I also see patients come back in ten or twelve years for a redo. I knew my outlook was bleak. I was absolutely desperate. I prayed every day, but who was I to expect God to hear my plea when there were so many others in far worse condition?

But God did answer my prayers. In October 2003, as I was driving home from work, I remembered that Dr. Rhodes had once worked a miracle for me with orthotics. So I drove to his office with hope in my heart that he could once again help me. Never in my wildest dreams did I imagine what a difference that day would make in my life. He told me, "I can give you orthotics, but I've got something far better than that for you now." I made an appointment for the very next day.

On October 15, 2003, I went to Dr. Rhodes for testing and began using his electrical stimulation device. He advised getting off the prednisone, hydrocodone and neurontin as quickly as I could. I knew I had to wean off the prednisone slowly, but I went off the hydrocodone and the neurontin immediately. They were not controlling the pain, and if getting them out of my system would allow the electrical treatments to work more effectively, I was willing to go for it. Then something incredible happened.

I had had no feeling in my feet for 2 years due to neuropathy caused by the arthritis, which had triggered vasculitis. The nerve pain was so bad I couldn't sleep. The sheets touching my feet, or wearing shoes or socks caused excruciating pain. It felt like all the bones in my feet were broken. I couldn't walk. It was horrible. The doctors had told me my condition was not reversible. But they were wrong.

On the third day of the treatments, I could feel water hit my feet. On the fourth day I had no pain in my wrist, had increased flexion in my left ankle, decreased swelling in my hands, feet, and knees. On the eighth day of treatment, I wrote in my journal. "VERY good day—easy walking, no pain until 6:30pm." **On the 11th day** I had my **first pain free day** for as long as I can remember!! I continued to improve. The electrical stimulation worked very well and very quickly on my arthritis.

On March 5, 2004 (4 months after starting the treatments), I had an appointment with my rheumatologist in San Antonio. Prior to going to that appointment, I had blood drawn for lab work. That lab work showed I was having a major inflammatory episode; however, I showed no clinical signs of inflammation. No joints were swollen and I had no pain. Proof that Dr. Rhodes' electrical therapy was working to control the arthritis symptoms!

Dr. Rhodes' electrical stimulation therapy has kept my arthritis symptoms at bay for three and a half years. The neuralgia from the neuropathy is also going away. Whereas three and a half years ago I had no feeling in my feet except for excruciating nerve pain, now the sensations in my feet are normal. I can feel everything: hot, cold, wet, soft, etc. There is still an area about the size of a quarter on my left foot where the nerves are still regenerating and that area can get my attention very quickly. The electrical treatments control the pain and soon the nerves should be regenerated to the point that that pain is also gone.

I am 60. I married my high school sweetheart when I was 19. We have been married 39 years, and Ed has been with me and loved me through all the ups and downs of this disease. I have had RA since I was six. In all that time, no doctor and no drug was able to stop the disease, but Dr. Rhodes and his electrical stimulation therapy had the disease under control in four months!

When I try to spread the word about Dr. Rhodes, I feel the way the disciples of Jesus must have felt. I know about this, I have experienced it and have seen other people experience it. I know it's the truth. I go out and tell people, but they don't believe me.

Dr. Rhodes' treatment is a miracle and I pray God blesses him as much as his treatment has blessed all of us he has helped.

~~~~~

Morgan Henry

She was in such pain she wanted to cut her leg off. She couldn't walk, couldn't think straight, and had no quality of life. And, she was facing life in a wheelchair.

Susan, Morgan's mother:

In May, 1998, when Morgan was 14, she sprained her left foot playing soccer. The injury seemed minor. Two months later, she sprained it again. This time the pain became intense and wouldn't let up. So we sought treatment. Morgan had two months of laser treatment in Dallas/Forth Worth in August and September of 1998. Then she had four sympathetic blocks in October and November of 1998 in Torrance, California. In addition, she tried acupuncture, physical therapy, psychotherapy, dance therapy, and various medications from October 1998 until May 1999. However, she was still in chronic pain.

Meanwhile, I had taken her to doctors all over California and called doctors around the country. One doctor thought she was faking. He told her if she wanted to quit soccer, she should just quit. Other doctors wanted to perform all kinds of invasive procedures on Morgan. One said he would give her ten spinal epidurals, one right after the other, without stopping. That seemed so drastic for a fourteen-year-old. I wanted a safe, non-invasive treatment for my daughter.

What troubled me most was the fear I saw in the doctors' eyes. I was going to pretty well-known experts, yet they had no confidence that they could help her. And they couldn't answer many of my questions, such as, "How many injections will it take?" or "How many procedures will it take?" They didn't know.

What were we to do? We couldn't give up because by this time my daughter's pain was escalating and spreading from her ankle up her leg. I was frantic to help her.

Then, I stumbled across the name of Dr. Rhodes. I even had access to a video in which some of his pain patients told their success stories. I was skeptical, but I got from Dr. Rhodes the names of some other patients who had been successfully treated and contacted them. Still I wasn't convinced. And then, the unimaginable happened. Morgan had an accident where a hammer fell on her left foot! I was scared out of my mind. Every little bump since that first injury just added to her pain. Later I believe that accident to be an act of God, trying to get us to Dr. Rhodes.

My worst fears were realized when the hammer incident threw Morgan into the worse kind of agony anyone can imagine. She was in such pain she wanted to cut her leg off. She couldn't walk, couldn't think straight, and had no quality of life. And, she was facing life in a wheelchair. I walked around the house and cried and cried and cried. Nothing has ruined my soul more than my daughter being sick. What was happening to us? Why did no one know how to treat my daughter's horrible pain condition?

I was desperate. I called Dr. Rhodes' office, still hesitant. He said, "There's a soccer mom here. I'll let you talk to her."

I had heard success stories from other patients I had previously called. I had watched the video with great skepticism. I had already taken Morgan to so many doctors who could not really help her. How could I subject her to another failed procedure? How could I give her hope once more only to have it snatched away again? But as a soccer mom, I trusted one of my own kind. It took another soccer mom, whose son was making remarkable progress, to convince me to give Dr. Rhodes a try. Morgan and I were in Corpus Christi within 3 days after the hammer accident.

We had already been flying back and forth from California to Dallas/Fort Worth for laser treatment. On the plane, we could not believe we had to return to Texas for more treatment. With all the doctors and hospitals in California, we were saying, what's up with Texas!

In Corpus Christi, we were driven by the hotel shuttle service to Dr. Rhodes' clinic. The driver said, "Oh, you're going to Dr. Rhodes. He's like a miracle man. I've never met him, but I drive patients to him all the time. Somebody was just here from Australia. She came on crutches and she left walking. That happens over and over." That gave me hope.

We arrived at Dr. Rhodes' clinic in January, 1999. I still wondered how a doctor in Texas could help Morgan when nobody else had been able to. But he was totally different from all other doctors we had seen. The first thing he said to Morgan was, "Just trust me. I will get you better." We had a strong belief that he was right. He inspired so much confidence, unlike the other doctors who got that horrified look on their faces because they didn't know what they were treating.

Dr. Rhodes had only one machine then. He was treating several other children when we were there, so everyone had to share the machine by taking turns using it. But that didn't matter because, eventually, we could all see our kids getting better.

However, because Morgan did not respond to the treatment immediately, she doubted that she'd get well. So Doc would circle each painful spot with a dark marker pen. Then he would work and work on just that spot. And he worked spot by spot, day after day, and the painful spots went away. He also encouraged the kids by setting up competitions to see who would improve the fastest. That really motivated them. Soon Morgan was walking with a smile on her face that would brighten anyone's day.

I would almost call Dr. Rhodes a healer. He did so much to treat the whole person, not just the disease. He made Morgan, the other kids at the clinic, and all the parents feel like family. He gave us so much time. We went to his house after office hours and hung out with him, his wife, and their kids.

In spite of everyone's best efforts, Morgan did not get well within 15 days as we had planned, so we extended. Doc said she had to have three pain free days before she could go home. We were relieved and so grateful when she was able to walk out of Dr. Rhodes' office pain free 30 days after our arrival. We returned to his clinic in April, 1999, for a tune up to get rid of any residual pain, but by the time she arrived in Corpus Christi, she felt great.

After that, Morgan resumed what was basically a normal life. Although there was no home STS machine then, Morgan did have a TENS unit and another small machine that she ran together with specific protocols from Doc. She used magnets to make the machines more effective. She also wore magnets during the day with high top tennis shoes for stability. In the shoes she wore orthotics, which had been custom made by Doc. The high top tennis shoes made quite a fashion statement in high school! She was mortified to wear them, but happy to be well, so she endured. Doc also sent special cream via overnight express when the pain was starting to build up and she became fearful. We would call him, he would talk to her, give her courage, mix a batch of special pain cream, and send it. It worked. She was usually feeling better by the time the cream arrived.

We realized even more how blessed we were to have learned of Dr. Rhodes when Morgan spoke at an RSD meeting. At that gathering, there were 100 to 150 people there, most of them in wheelchairs, all seeking help for their terrible pain. Equally chilling were the many references to RSD sufferers whose names were followed by the phrase "in memory of" because those patients had died. That's when I realized what a real miracle man Dr. Rhodes is.

As for Morgan, she resumed playing soccer in high school and played in college for a year. Now she plays college club soccer. At age 22, she is doing great.

After our experience, I always tell patients who go to Dr. Rhodes that they MUST believe that they will get better. That is the most important thing they can do. And when they meet Dr. Rhodes, it's easy for them to believe they will be healed. He's that good.

Susan Henry
Manhattan Beach, California

~~~~~

M.

Holland

For me, surgery worked like an explosion that triggered intense nerve pain that wouldn't go away.

I was interested in staying healthy, so I regularly did indoor rowing and biking. One day, on November 19, 1999, I hit my knee under a table. It wasn't a big injury. I developed what you would call normal pain afterward. However, the pain didn't stop. So in May of 2000, I had what they call exploratory keyhole surgery to see what was wrong. That means they make a very small hole instead of a big incision. Even so, it can take a year to two to completely heal.

I know now I shouldn't have had that operation. But I didn't know it then. Two weeks after I had it, I went to an orthopedic surgeon on crutches to have the scars examined. A month later, terrible nerve pain developed and did not let up. My knee felt as if it had a band around it. The color changed. I had burning pain. I had to walk slowly. I went back to the doctor. He is one of the most famous knee surgeons in Holland. He said I could get that kind of pain only from a real operation.

It's so strange that doctors do not know about this kind of pain reaction. They need to know about it so they can tell you the risks of having an operation. For me, surgery worked like an explosion that triggered intense nerve pain that wouldn't go away. I didn't understand what I had. My life changed drastically. I felt tired. Friends didn't visit often. I spent a lot of time crying from hurting. So much of my time revolved around my pain and trying to get rid of it. Some doctors who didn't know what I had dismissed my complaints. One gave me the name of an anesthesiologist who gave me some cream that smelled like onions. It didn't work. I had IV's and medication. One doctor congratulated me when he told me I didn't have RSD. Everybody told me something different. Then my pain went up my leg and into my other knee. I was in a panic.

Finally, a physical therapist diagnosed me. She said she could have helped me if I had gone to her right after the injury. But she worked on me anyway to see if she could give me some relief. From July, 2000 until August 2001, I had 100 connective tissue massages. They were a type of deep rubbing of my leg to help the blood and oxygen flow. It helped, and I learned to do it myself. After a treatment I could walk a little bit. That provided me a little recovery, but then it stopped. I had to look somewhere else for help.

So I tried the Internet. I found more than 400 websites about RSD. Some were hotels, spas, and resorts trying to attract business and offer people a good time. The rest told about

RSD but offered no cure. The descriptions of RSD were different from one site to another. If these people knew what they were talking about, all the sites should have given basically the same information. I felt sure Japan would have some good treatments. But they treat it with brain surgery. I called a doctor I found on an Italian website. He used a hyperbaric chamber, like those used for divers. He'd had to close the clinic after an accident had killed some patients. I was discouraged, at best. And I was desperate.

Then I found Dr. Rhodes' website. His was the only one offering a real solution. Could he be right? His site was encouraging, but Texas is a long way from Holland. Would a trip to the United States be worth it? Before I could decide, I wanted to know if he'd treated patients from Europe. So I checked with him and learned he was treating someone from England. She had suffered for 6 years before she got to Dr. Rhodes. He said he'd never had a patient as bad off as she was. She stayed at his clinic six weeks and later returned to England very satisfied with her results. Before she went to Texas, she had checked with a patient in Australia who had been to Dr. Rhodes and was happy with the outcome.

This news was encouraging. My husband and I decided to make the trip to Dr. Rhodes' clinic. I took a little valium to help me make the flight. When I arrived, my pain level was 8. Dr. Rhodes treated me and answered my questions, and I improved. I returned to Holland in much better shape and used the machine regularly. I still had some pain, but nothing like before. I could walk much farther and carry out most of my usual activities for the first time since I developed RSD. I was so grateful.

Then almost five years later, I learned that Dr. Rhodes had new methods that could help me even more than the first time. On my original trip, he used similar frequencies on the machine on almost everybody. And he had to try different protocols to see which worked best. But now he could test for the best frequency setting for the individual patient and could test for the best protocols to use on that patient. So he was getting better results faster. My husband and I decided to go back to Texas for the enhanced quality of medical treatment.

When I arrived in Corpus Christi in April, 2006, my overall pain level was seven. That night before my first office visit, I suffered from severe cramps in my left foot (I have RSDS in my left knee, you know). The next day, Dr. Rhodes tested me for several protocols and treated me, and after three days the cramps totally disappeared.

I have had migraines about once a month since I was a teenager. While I was in Corpus Christi I suffered from a severe attack for which I brought injections that I give myself. The injections work well, but every needle through the skin makes RSD worse. So back home I would use the machine to take care of that side effect. When I informed Dr. Rhodes about this condition, he gave me another protocol and he advised me to eat something after the treatment. The result was that I did not use any medicine for the migraine attack during my stay. Back home I had one attack, but less severe and less frequent. His machine is helping.

Another interesting thing is that flying is bad for RSDS patients, as Dr. Rhodes told me. Therefore, he gave me a special flight protocol, which I had to use three days before departure and for three days after arrival home. The trip left me hardly able to walk when I got off after twelve hours on the plane. So I used the special protocols for flying. After a few days my condition was as good as it had been in Corpus Christi. And I had left there after twelve days with my pain level down to two or three.

As of this writing, my pain level is two during the day, in the evening about four (when I do too much walking). In other words, the new approach Dr. Rhodes is using works better for me.

My husband and I don't panic anymore since we know Dr. Rhodes and his treatment.

~~~~~~

Donna

Before I went to Dr. Rhodes, I had ice put on my foot in therapy.
It felt like a blowtorch.

I injured myself in 1996. I was playing a lot of tennis and had some problems with the bottom of one foot. After a match, I yanked my tennis shoe off too quickly and tore a tendon in my left foot. The pain and incapacity were so bad that I began a round of going to doctors. Basically, they told me, "Keep doing what you're doing." So I continued my daily activities the best that I could. But the pain persisted. Finally, a doctor put me in a boot-like cast.

Before long, the pain escalated. It was excruciating. I was given therapy and told I needed surgery. In therapy, I had ice put on my foot. It felt like a blowtorch. I tried various doctors, hoping someone could help me. I saw three orthopedists, one podiatrist, and a Chinese doctor in Fort Worth. They all gave me different advice: surgery, injections, therapy. I rejected the surgery and injections. The therapy didn't help a bit.

I felt so frustrated. The pain was searing, relentless, debilitating. I could no longer walk. I had to use a wheel chair. I was desperate. My normal life of active days, plans for the future, and zest for living had become a tortured quest for relief from a type of burning pain that felt like being held captive in Hades. Somewhere in the midst of this nightmare, Dr. Rhodes' name came up. I was told he had a machine that could resolve my pain. It wouldn't involve surgery, injections, or anything painful. It was totally non-invasive. At first I was skeptical. I didn't want to believe it because I was afraid it wouldn't work.

One day I saw a TV show about RSD. A man suffering from it was in such pain that he shot his foot. I knew what he was experiencing. I didn't know if that's what I had, but I really related to what he said. Not long after that my defenses were so worn down by the constant torment in my foot that I picked up the phone and called Dr. Rhodes. In tears, I explained my situation, outlined the procedures the other doctors had wanted me to undergo, and told him I had all my medical records, if that would help.

Dr. Rhodes replied that the invasive therapies the other doctors had suggested— surgery, injections—were the worst things I could have done. They would have only made matters worse. He said he liked the challenge of difficult cases. My condition sounded like what he'd been having success with, so he thought he could help me. I didn't want to get my hopes up, but I went to his clinic to check it out. While there, I saw patients from out of state who had come in wheel chairs and walked out three months later. That blew me away. So I agreed to have him treat me. When I'd get discouraged because it seemed to take so long, those recovered patients gave me the determination to stick with it.

Dr. Rhodes treated me for three to four months, two to three times a week. At the end of that time, I still had some pain, but he said I didn't need to come back because his testing showed that I was clear of the underlying cause of the pain. He explained that, after the sympathetic nervous system is normalized, it takes up to six months for the body to completely heal itself. Dr. Rhodes didn't have a home machine then, and I was fearful that I'd relapse. I asked him if the pain would return again in full force. He said that, as of then, it hadn't returned in anybody he'd treated as far as he knew.

In the fall of 1997, Dr. Rhodes released me from his clinic. I was free of my wheel chair but still had some mild pain, which lasted for about six months. During that time, I had to be careful of the shoes I wore, so I lived in tennis shoes with orthotics Dr. Rhodes had made for me. I gradually got better. Dr. Rhodes had told me, "The more you exercise, the better." So I walked regularly and took up tennis again in January, 1998. Six months after my last treatment, I realized that I no longer favored my left foot. I resumed wearing high heels. The pain had completely resolved. And it has remained that way until this day, eight years later. As a matter of fact, I am in the middle of training for a dance contest and have been practicing four hours a day. The minor aches I have gotten from that intense workout are the normal result of overdoing it. They are not RSD. However, if I had one of Dr. Rhodes' machines, I would use it to take care of those little pains, too. After what he did for me, I totally believe in his machine. And I'm grateful that I found out about Dr. Rhodes before I resorted to invasive forms of treatment that might have done permanent damage.

Update, August, 2006

I did just fine until 2006, when I was highly involved in dancing and more dancing, as I mentioned above. I kept up a very heavy routine of practice, putting tremendous strain on my feet. As I said in the previous paragraph, I began to have some pain. But I danced through it all, which is the worst thing I could have done.

Anyone who has ever had RSD should never ignore pain. Catching it early means faster recovery. But I fooled around. I didn't want to admit what was happening or give in to it. That was a mistake.

Finally, when I realized I was getting worse and not better, I went back to Dr. Rhodes. Although the pain wasn't as bad as the first time he treated me, testing showed the RSD was back. He began protocols and then ran an MRI. He could hardly believe the results. I had torn the same tendon as I had back in 1999. He didn't know how I could have kept going and have done so much in that condition.

He could treat the pain, but I had to stay off my feet, then use crutches, a cane, and finally wear special shoes to allow the tendon to heal. And I bought one of his machines for home use.

It looks like I'll always have a tendency to have tendon problems. My father has them, and his mother did, too. She also had red legs that burned like crazy. I realize now that was a form of RSD. So it also runs in my family.

I am becoming more and more active again. That means I run Dr. Rhodes' machine less because I'm so busy. I keep my pain level down to a one or two most days, unless I really engage in a lot of activity. Then it may go to a three the day after. If I'd take it easier, I'd heal faster. But I love activities like water skiing, tennis, and dancing. And now that I have Dr. Rhodes' machine, I can treat myself on my own schedule or put up with minor pain if I decide not to take time to run the protocols regularly.

I returned to normal before. I expect to again. It just may take a little longer since I like to keep on the move. I am grateful to Dr. Rhodes that I have that choice. With his machine on hand, if pain crops up, I can treat it right away and not let it escalate.

~~~~~

Megan

Silsbee, Texas

The doctors talked to us about amputating Megan's leg. A better possibility would be to paralyze her from the waist down. She'd spend the rest of her life in a wheelchair, but she might beat the pain—maybe. The thought horrified us. We were frantic.

This story is written by Megan and her family from Silsbee, Texas, to share with others an understanding of the pain and agony of RSD and the wonderful treatment she received from Dr. Donald Alan Rhodes and his staff in Corpus Christi, Texas.

When Megan was eight years old, she broke her right foot while jumping on a trampoline. It was in a cast and seemed to heal okay but was always weak. On May 13, 2001, two days after her tenth birthday, she sprained her right foot as she stepped out of our camper trailer. We took her to the Bone and Joint Clinic, where an x-ray showed no broken bones. They diagnosed it as RSD. She was referred to a pain specialist in Houston, Texas.

Meanwhile, within three weeks the pain had moved from her foot to the top of her leg and was so intense she could not bear any weight on it and was on crutches. Her treatment consisted of five lidocaine pain blocks and pool therapy, which did not work. By now Megan was in a wheelchair, unable to walk even with the aid of crutches. The pain was so bad she couldn't tolerate anything touching her leg and foot, not even the sheets. She could not take a tub bath, so she had to be pan bathed. She couldn't stand to pass by the air conditioner return air vent because the breeze hurt her so badly. She felt every bump and vibration while riding in the car. She was on strong pain medication but still was in constant pain. She got no relief, none. Megan described her pain as being struck by lightning with a blowtorch put on her foot and leg.

The doctor said the next step was to put an epidural pump in her spine, which would shoot pain medication to her right leg constantly. This was tried for two weeks with no results. At this time Megan was getting worse. Her leg was discolored, and the foot was drawing inward.

At that point the doctors talked to our family about Megan's quality of life. Obviously, they held out no hope for a cure. Amputation was a choice, but it was a long shot. Soldiers in the Civil War had tried it, only to continue in pain. A better possibility would be to paralyze her from the waist down. She'd spend the rest of her life in a wheelchair, but she might beat the pain--maybe. The thought horrified us. We were frantic.

Then the doctor said he could implant a morphine pump in her spine to see if that would work. He couldn't guarantee it would. That option certainly was preferable to paralyzing her. We had to do something. She was crying and screaming in pain. Sometimes she would pass out when she could no longer tolerate it. We had a home health nurse coming out every day. Megan couldn't think, she felt confused; she couldn't read. Obviously, she couldn't attend school. Her life was a nightmare.

The morphine pump procedure was to be scheduled the week of August 6, 2001. Megan's mom phoned the Houston doctor's office on August 1 to see on which day the procedure had been scheduled. She was told that the doctor had gone on vacation and would be out all week. This made her furious. But it turned out to be a blessing and was part of the miracle that we had been praying for.

Megan's grandmother had done research on the Internet and found Dr. Rhodes in Corpus Christi, Texas. He specialized in RSD and had success in treating it. Previously, Megan's mom had thought that doctors in Houston, which she considered the medical Mecca of the world, would have the most up to date medical knowledge, techniques, and procedures. However, after finding out the Houston doctor had left on vacation, she got the phone number of Dr. Rhodes' clinic in Corpus Christi and made an appointment for Friday, August 3, 2001. We left for Corpus Christi on August 2. Megan was in extreme pain and felt every bump and vibration from the car on the way. Corpus Christi is very windy, and the wind was extremely painful to Megan on our arrival.

Megan went into Dr. Rhodes' office at 8:00 a.m. on August 3, 2001, in extreme pain. Her mom took her to a treatment room and returned to the front office to take care of paper work. Forty minutes later she returned to the treatment room. Megan was sitting up, rubbing her leg. She looked at her mom with an expression of wonder. "Mom," she said. "The doctor used something called the magnetron on me. The pain is gone." We couldn't believe it. After all that time, all she had been through, all that the other doctors had tried, we finally had an answer. We all just bawled.

The magnetron is a machine Dr. Rhodes uses when the patient is too sensitive to touch to tolerate electrodes. After that initial treatment, he treated Megan with his regular machine. Dr. Rhodes gradually took Megan off all the strong medications. She was out of the wheelchair and on crutches after five treatments. She walked without crutches after 8 treatments. She had a total of twenty treatments, and we purchased a machine to take home for her to use.

Megan remained pain free for four months. She was active, back in school, and taking band. Then, she began to feel the vibrations of the music and asking for pain medication. The pain became constant, but it wasn't as intense as before. So we took her back to Dr. Rhodes. She stayed only seven days the second time. She felt better the first night after we got there.

The site of the pain had changed somewhat, so Dr. Rhodes gave her different protocols. And he fixed her again. He said she might be one of the people who need to use the machine indefinitely. By February 2006, Megan had spent two years as a cheerleader in middle school with only minor problems and was doing well. She continues to use the machine as a precaution. If she feels a little twinge here and there, she hooks herself up and takes a treatment. She uses it maybe once a month now. Otherwise, she remains pain free.

Today, Megan would be paralyzed and in a wheel chair if we'd stayed with our doctors. Her life would be radically different. Instead, Dr. Rhodes gave us back our happy little girl. We are so grateful to him. In our opinion, he worked a miracle for our Megan.

~~~~~~

Christy

Christy developed pain in her right shoulder at 2:00 p.m. By 7:00 p.m. her arm had turned black. She couldn't eat, she couldn't sleep, she was in terrible shape. I was afraid she was going to die. If she lived, the pain would have disabled her for life.

Christy's father:

Christy was 21 and a senior in nursing school. I was proud that she chose to enter the medical profession. She was doing well until she had a car wreck. She hit a deer on the highway, and it crashed through her windshield and landed in the front seat, where it injured her right arm. The wreck totaled the car. She was lucky to be alive.

We naturally expected her to need time to recover. However, she began to have symptoms in her arm that one doctor thought could be the blood vessels shutting down.

About six weeks after the accident, Christy developed pain in her right shoulder at 2:00 p.m. By 7:00 p.m. her arm had turned black. I took her to the emergency room. A physician there, whose daughter had suffered from RSD, recognized the symptoms. He gave Christy the standard treatment at that time, ganglion blocks and narcotics. The color and warmth returned to her arm, but the pain persisted.

Then the doctor knocked her out with oxycontin. That was followed by a morphine drip. Nothing helped. She couldn't eat, she couldn't sleep, she was in terrible shape. I was afraid she was going to die. If she lived, the pain would have disabled her for life.

During Christy's hospitalization, a doctor told us about his daughter, who had been treated by Dr. Rhodes. The daughter, who had been disabled by RSD, could now run and play sports. As a doctor myself, I was skeptical. Dr. Rhodes was a podiatrist. I had a wall of opposition because of who he was. But I was also desperate. So we went to Corpus Christi. After the first treatment, Christy slept all night for the first time in two weeks. She continued treatments with Dr. Rhodes and left pain free.

She returned to nursing school, got her license, and now works as a pediatric nurse.

To this day I don't understand how Dr. Rhodes does what he does. But that doesn't matter. What does matters is that it worked for my daughter.

Christy:

I don't remember much about my eleven days in the hospital after the wreck with the deer. I was in so much pain and on so much medication that it's a blur. But I know it was terrible for my family.

I had no idea that at age 21 I was a candidate for such an awful disease. However, I have since learned that people who develop RSD often have previous conditions associated with it. In my case, I had a lot of pain in my feet when I was younger and often cried because of it. I vomited a lot during my life and had headaches and nausea. So the encounter with the deer just happened to be the trigger that set off full-blown RSD.

At Dr. Rhodes' clinic, the first day of treatments produced wonderful results. The pain vanished. Dr. Rhodes explained that I needed follow up protocols on a daily basis to keep the pain at bay until my body could heal itself. So, I was at his clinic for 15 days to get me on the path to remission. I've had two flare ups that required a trip back to Dr. Rhodes, one at age 22, when I stayed seven days, and another at age 26, when I stayed five days. I was concerned when I became pregnant that I might have problems, but Dr. Rhodes developed special protocols for me, and everything went fine.

As for home treatments over the long term, I have one of Dr. Rhodes' machines that I keep under my bed. I use it to get back to normal only when I have symptoms. Since as a pediatric nurse I work 12 and 14-hour shifts, I need to be in great health to handle everything. And I can.

Dr. Rhodes has given me back my life. He is absolutely wonderful. Without him, I don't know where I'd be now.

~~~~~~

Sarah

I developed extreme pain in October 2001. I deteriorated so much that by December I didn't have enough strength to lift a glass of water.

Summer, 2002

Dear Dr. Rhodes and Staff,

Thank you very much for what you have done for me.

Before I got sick with RSDS, I was golfing and very committed to my schoolwork. I was having some trouble with my knees, so in September 2001, a physician and a physical therapist both recommended taping my knees. We tried the taping at home ourselves and at a physical therapist facility. This is the only indication of an injury that I could come up with that led to RSDS.

Then, I developed extreme pain in October 2001. I deteriorated so much that by December I didn't have enough strength to lift a glass of water. By Christmas the pain had moved to all four of my limbs and jaw. I could no longer use my hands to eat. Basically, I just screamed all day.

My parents and I were desperate. They took me everywhere for help. I saw fifteen different doctors. I went to the Mayo Clinic, St. Louis Children's Hospital, and all over Central Illinois. Every doctor had a different diagnosis, never RSDS. We asked the last doctor I saw if it could be RSDS. He said no, because it was not confined to one limb. However, he decided to treat me as if I had RSDS. His plan was to up my ultram and neurontin every week until the pain was under control. I was on other medication, too. Nothing helped.

In January 2002, my pediatrician recommended that we go to Connecticut to see one of the nation's top doctors and a medical team that specializes in RSDS. It took us six weeks to get in. Three days before we were supposed to leave, we got a call from the doctor. He told us that they were not going to help us.

Believe it or not, that devastating call was the best thing that could have happened. The day after that call, my mom saw Dr. Rhodes' website on the Internet. She called him the next day. We got in the following week. I was there for six and a half weeks. I got off all pain and nerve medication. Dr. Rhodes has given me back my life. I was able to go back and finish the school year at home with a tutor while getting high honors. I plan to go to school this next school year.

Thank you,
Sarah, Age 13
Groveland, Il

~~~~~~

Joe

My brother-in-law lost his foot due to gangrene. Eventually, he died from the effects of diabetes. A friend had such bad diabetic ulcers that he had to have his foot amputated. My eyes were deteriorating from diabetes. I had ten or more laser surgeries on them. I had diabetic ulcers on my legs. Was I next for some terrible outcome? I was frantic.

When I learned a local doctor was looking for diabetic patients for a medical study, I enrolled immediately. My brother-in-law had lost his foot. He had gangrene. He died from the effects of diabetes. A friend has such bad diabetic ulcers that he had to have his foot amputated. As for me, my eyes were deteriorating from diabetes. I had ten or more laser surgeries on them. I was going blind. I knew people like me who had eye problems from diabetes and suddenly lost their vision. I didn't want to depend on people to take me where I needed to go. I dreaded what was in store for me. Really, it was worse than that. I was frantic.

Because my diabetes was so bad, I was on insulin. But it didn't keep my blood sugar under control. And I had all these health problems as a result. I had real bad peripheral neuropathy for ten years. I could hardly walk because my feet were so painful. I had shoulder and hip pain at the level of nine to ten. I had gained 100 pounds and was up to 300 pounds. I was tired all the time. I had large, deep ulcers on my legs that my wife cleaned and dressed every day. It always took six or seven weeks for them to heal. The doctor wanted to graft skin over the ulcers because he said that was the only way to fix them. I asked him, "What are you going to do about the places on my body where you remove the skin to put over the ulcers?"

I figured I had nothing to lose by getting in a study about diabetes. But I had no idea the results would be so good. After a week, my pain level went down to three or four, and I could walk. The ulcers on my legs healed in one week. The increased blood circulation to the ulcers made the difference. My eyes got better. My need for insulin started going down. When the study is over, I expect to feel even better than I do now.

Because of Dr. Rhodes' treatments, I have a much better quality of life. I am able to get up, move around, and I can see. I like to fish and play golf with my grandson, and now I have the energy to do those things.

If you have diabetes and you don't try Dr. Rhodes' machine, I would say you're foolish. It's not like getting on medicine that can harm your body. When you begin to heal, you need to take good care of your body and run the machine regularly. That's the secret. And if problems crop up, you need to go back for a tune up.

These treatments, I'm sold on them.

~~~~~~

Sara

Clayton, California

A lot of people thought Sara was faking or exaggerating her pain. Even some doctors didn't believe her. We were desperate.

Carol, Sara's mother:

I'm the mother of a close knit family. What affects one of us affects us all. When Sara was in pain, we were all in pain. It was especially hard on Sara's twin sister. Imagine if you can that your life is going along as you would expect. Then, out of the blue, everything is turned upside down. That's what happened to us.

Sara was a swimmer. At the age of 14, she somehow hit her hand, maybe on the pool. She developed intense pain in her entire right arm. She was put in a cast. Her fingers swelled up. Before we got to Dr. Rhodes many years later, she'd been to more than fifteen different doctors. She underwent acupuncture, nerve blocks, ganglion blocks, and chiropractic treatments. During one procedure, a needle punctured her lung. She was so desperate to eliminate the pain that she told one doctor to cut off her arm. If she got any pain relief, it was temporary. It took a year to get a diagnosis of RSD.

Finally, Sara had an operation to implant a nerve stimulator. She turned it on and regulated it with a remote control. She kept it running 24 hours a day. She wore it for a year and felt good. Finally, she no longer needed to turn it on, but the doctor left it in for six months longer before removing it just in case she had a relapse. She thought she was cured. She did fine for years.

Then at age 24, she cut a finger on her right hand on a picture frame. That triggered RSD a week later. She developed stinging, burning, just like the first time she was in pain. She couldn't move her fingers. She lay around and cried. She was given narcotic medications and neurontin. Nothing helped.

Three months after the RSD returned, she had another operation to have a nerve stimulator implanted. It helped again. She got off all pain medication. Six months later, the stimulator broke down twice and was repaired, requiring more surgery. Then one day during a walk, a wire from the device pierced the skin in her back. So the unit was removed and a third one scheduled to be implanted.

Instead of using the typical pathway for implanting the stimulator, the surgeon had to go through her neck because of scar tissue from the previous operations. That made the surgery very difficult. Three hours into the operation, the doctor almost quit. He couldn't get the implant in. He talked to us before proceeding and decided to cut away some bone to get the device installed. Then he threaded the wires in through her spinal column. When he finished, he wasn't sure how effective it would be since the unit didn't have the same contact area as before.

Sara was in a lot of pain from the surgery, but she got some relief from the RSD for a couple of months. She healed from the operation, but the stimulator had to be programmed to its maximum levels, and she had to meet with the programmer twice a week to make adjustments. Then we learned that scar tissue was growing around the device, which changed the efficiency of the stimulator.

Sara suffered even though she used the stimulator plus heavy medication for about a year. She would have to go to the emergency room several times a week for injections of demerol.

Finally, the pain doctor referred us to a physical therapist who had trained with Dr. Rhodes and who used his machine to treat pain. However, when it didn't help, the therapist recommended that we take Sara to be treated by Dr. Rhodes himself. She'd worked on other patients whose pain was beyond her ability, and they had returned home from Dr. Rhodes' clinic marvelously better.

By this time, Sara's pain had skyrocketed to unbelievable intensity. One doctor had told her, "You're going to have to live with the pain." She hurt so badly and was on so much medication that she'd turned into a complete zombie.

It was frustrating that a lot of people thought Sara was faking or exaggerating her pain. Even some doctors didn't believe her. We were desperate. Our daughter's life had been shattered, we'd done everything within our power to help her, we'd taken her everywhere for treatment, we'd seen her through the ups and downs of deteriorating until she had no quality of life left, and there were no avenues left to us.

Unless...

What convinced us to travel to Texas was a video of a doctor whose daughter had been successfully treated by Dr. Rhodes. It seemed unreal that a machine that didn't hurt, didn't invade the body, and had already failed in the hands of a therapist could perform the magic on Sara that no one else had been able to perform. But we had to give it a try. And so we did.

Carol and Keith, Sara's Parents:

August 22, 2002

Dear Dr. Rhodes:

You are a miracle worker.

There are no words to express the gratitude we feel for what you have done for our daughter Sara and for our whole family. To see Sara off all her medications and enjoying life again is indescribable. I always knew it would happen because you would never give up on her. You give so much of yourself to each of your patients, and I will never forget how you were always there for us.

You have a gift to give to the whole world. Your knowledge of RSD and your continued pursuit to let everyone who is suffering with RSD know that there is hope and that your machine and protocols can give them back their lives is just waiting to be heard.

Sara comes from a very close family, and the change this has made in all our lives continues to grow. Sara is always laughing and smiling and not always sleeping her life away like she used to. She gets up early, stays up, and has the energy to do things. It is amazing. I used to be afraid every day because I never knew what Sara's pain level was going to be and how we could cope with it. She was lost, as was her whole family, in this horrible disease. Now I embrace each new day and celebrate the gift you have given us by giving us back our daughter.

I feel blessed to have found you. Your positive attitude and commitment to succeed when most doctors would have given up on our Sara made this happen. I remember the first day we got there and you said, "I know I can get you off your medications and pain free. I won't give up on you. I despise defeat and don't allow it to happen." You had the gentle strength that Sara needed and counted on. It was important for her to know you would not give up on her. You listened to all of her concerns and counseled her through the bumps in the road. You gave her the strength to do her part so you could do your part.

So much of what I am feeling is hard to put into words. I am soooooo grateful and I am smiling and laughing all the time now, too!!!

You have given us the greatest gift of all, our daughter Sara back.

Thank you,
Carol and Keith

Sara:

My name is Sara. A little over two months from now, I will be turning 30 and getting married. A little more than two years ago, I could barely plan ahead a few hours because of the almost constant debilitating pain I suffered.

I suffered from something called Reflex Sympathetic Nerve Dystrophy, which is a complex condition where the nerves are certain there is danger in a certain part of the body, sending all sorts of pain signals to the brain, even though there is no discernable injury to the body. In my case, the condition started from a cut on a finger of my right hand, and long after that injury healed, my body was still processing pain that felt as if my arm were on fire all the time. Although this condition is becoming better known in the medical community, it's very hard to treat effectively, because even if one therapy works for a while, the condition can circumvent the treatment and come back stronger than ever. Before I found out about Dr. Donald Rhodes, I had consulted more than 20 doctors in California alone. They tried physical therapy, acupuncture, nerve blocks (one of which punctured my lungs), casting my right arm, biofeedback, neuro-feedback, chiropractic treatments, watsu water therapy, three different spinal cord stimulator implants, and five separate surgeries resulting from complications due to the stimulators. Throughout all of this, I was on a seemingly endless stream of medications. Just the ones I remember include neurontin, vicodin, darvocet, oxycontin, effexor, trazadone, demerol, morphine, and a demerol patch I had to wear every day. There were also innumerable trips to the emergency room every other week or so because my pain was so severe I needed a demerol injection. Between the pain and the medication, I was like a zombie. It was very strange because in some ways I was so strung out from the medication and the pain that I felt disconnected from almost everything normal, barely able to take care of the smallest, most mundane aspects of my life and health care. But because the pain was so severe, even though I was checked out emotionally a lot of the time, I was deeply connected to my pain, and completely unable to relax and feel any sense of comfort from all the treatments they were trying. The only solution my latest doctor could come up with was to increase my pain killers, despite the ridiculously high level of medication I was already on and the lack of relief it provided.

Had anyone looked at me during this time, they would have been completely puzzled about why I was so debilitated by pain. It was difficult explaining it to people. My family was unbelievably supportive, with my parents especially doing everything they could to help me. My fiancé, who was my boyfriend at the time, often had to take care of me as if I was a child. My mother became an expert on my condition, scouring the country for a miracle that would end my misery and give me my life back.

Little did I know it when my Mom and I packed off to Corpus Christi, Texas, but Dr. Rhodes was going to be my miracle. From the minute we arrived at his clinic, I knew there was something different about his practice from those of all the other doctors I had seen. It wasn't necessarily that he was more skilled; in fact, I had seen some incredibly talented and sympathetic physicians over the years. In part it was the obvious passion Dr. Rhodes had for treating the patients who came to him for help. He knew that for many of us he was our last hope, and he took seriously the despair of people in my position that feared they would never be free of pain. He told me right away that he thought he could help me. I was hardly optimistic, but I was willing to do whatever it took.

It was the middle of the summer in one of the hottest, most humid parts of the country. I couldn't stand the air conditioning because the feel of the breeze moving over my skin was enough to push me over the edge. My poor mother endured three months of stifling heat with no air conditioning, placing me in cool baths and tending to me along with Dr. Rhodes and all of his assistants and nurses. At the center of his treatment were an incredible intuition and intelligence, an unlimited well of personal compassion, and an innovative STS Dynatronic Machine, which was both non-invasive and non-toxic to the patient. The first thing he told me was that he was going to have to wean me off of the painkillers I was on, explaining that unless I was off the medication that he could not treat the pain effectively. He used the machine for part of this process, but a lot of it involved old-fashioned suffering as my body adjusted to the lack of medication and the increased pain levels in its absence.

There were moments when I felt I couldn't do it or that it wasn't worth more suffering, even if it was short term. Every time my resolve failed, Dr, Rhodes was there with the right thing to say and the understanding necessary to get me through to the next moment. He never flagged in his encouragement and support. He told me I could talk to him any time, that he would be available to me 24 hours a day, 7 days a week. There was no concern that was too small; he took seriously everything I said and felt, and when I wanted to quit, he gave me the strength and the desire to go on. The absolute conviction he had in his machine and in his therapy kept me going. Working with him was like stepping into the most secure, comforting space, where even though I was sometimes in misery, I became more and more certain that things would change, things would get better.

Truly, the hardest part of my treatment was getting all the pain medication out of my system. As this process wore on, though, I started having more and more moments of clarity and optimism. Dr. Rhodes was firm in his conviction that I had to get off the medication and unwavering in his belief that I would get better.

Dr. Rhodes treated me for three months. We had our ups and downs during that time, but by the time I was ready to return home to California, I was able to leave behind me years of horrendous pain, as well as an increasingly strong pessimism and a small duffle bag chock full of prescription medication. I came home with so much more, including hope for a normal future, the ability to do innumerable small things that had seemed monumental before, a small STS Dynatronic Machine to use on a daily basis, and a friend, mentor, and cheerleader for life in Dr. Rhodes.

I have been pain free for more than two years now. Each day I get farther away from that woman who was (barely) walking around in a drug induced stupor, totally unable to see past my haze of pain. Now I can go through days at a time without even thinking about those dark days, and even mixed in with those memories are all the moments of compassionate support Dr. Rhodes gave me. I tried to thank him once for giving me my life back, and all he would say to me was, "You always had it, but now it's what you make of it." You see, Dr. Rhodes doesn't have the time to bask in anyone's lavish praise, because he's too busy devoting every minute of every day to giving his patients the gifts of his compassion and expertise, and ultimately, of their future.

As I said before, I have met many talented and dedicated doctors over the years, but Dr. Rhodes is truly in a class by himself, and to me he exemplifies everything that is most noble and most profound about medicine--he helps people in the most humble way so that they can reach their highest potential. I think of him sometimes in the midst of my wedding plans, marveling at the fact that my life is so normal now, and how wonderful, how extraordinary normal can be.

Carol:

February 22, 2006

Dear Patricia,

I am delighted that you are writing a book on Dr. Rhodes.

Sara is doing great!!! She got married June 25, 2005, and will be finishing college this June with her degree, something she was unable to do until Dr. Rhodes entered her life.

She doesn't use the machine anymore, but I would really be interested in the new upgrades Dr. Rhodes has. I do get informed on what is going on because I am friends with some of his patients.

Our family is doing great. It is amazing how much Sara's pain free life has increased our whole family's sense of well being and happiness. You remember Sara is an identical twin, so her condition was very hard on her twin sister, Lisa, as well as on the rest of the family. Sara married her boyfriend she had during her illness. As we have all come to realize, it had really taken its toll on her husband. Their relationship is so wonderful and they are so happy now, it's hard to remember how awful it used to be when she was always in pain.

We feel blessed to have made the trip to Dr. Rhodes. We will never forget him.

Our journey to regain Sara from the depths of her painful existence led us to meet many wonderful people. Dr. Rhodes is a shining example of a giving and caring heart. He always made us feel safe and sure that he would always be there for Sara. I knew he would heal her and he did!

I am sure the book you are writing about him will be a much deserved tribute to his life of giving to others.

Carol:

June 4, 2006

Sara is married now and just graduated from College (yesterday). We are so proud of her!

Sara and her twin sister Lisa are both pregnant and expecting within a week of one another so you can see Sara is living her life to the fullest now and we thank Dr. Rhodes for that.

~~~~~~

A Glimpse into My Journal

The pain of RSD was unfathomable. There were guttural screams coming from the depths of my very core being from which I had never heard.

My words are written with devotion to my husband who lives with my conditions, through me, each and every day of his life. He has been thrown more curve balls, fast balls, high balls, low balls, you name them and he has hit them all, home runs each time, never walking, not once.

My words are also written in memory of my godfather (1926-2006) who passed away during my most recent visit to Dr. Rhodes.

I had been suffering from illnesses for years, which slowly started to manifest themselves necessitating the need for me to gather a team of specialists to care for my problems. I always do my best to exercise due diligence in managing my health care by communicating to each of these doctors, with whom I share a special bond, what was going on outside of their areas of expertise. At the time I had no idea my life was about to implode. I was sailing on a ship at sea, a passenger with a crew, yet I had no captain to chart the course and light the way. Then there came the day when my body was slammed by a huge wave of chronic pain known as Reflex Sympathetic Dystrophy Syndrome (RSDS) and under the bigger umbrella Autonomic Nervous System Dysfunction (ANSD). After trial and error a couple of times I found my captain in Dr. Donald Rhodes, D.P.M., P.A. The advantage he has, based on my experience, is that he knows bits and pieces about a multitude of specialties that enable him to have a unique perspective of an individual that is different from the eyes of a specialist. Dr. Rhodes treats causes and not just symptoms and encourages an individual to take charge of their health care. It is a big step, a leap of faith to go from traditional medicine to cutting edge technology offered by no one else that I have come across. When your body is wracked with so much pain making that decision, you would think, would be an easy one. But I was torn emotionally because my doctors have never heard of this Dr. Rhodes. He was not affiliated with some big name clinic in some big city. At the same time at some point I had to become what I consider selfish and put my needs first. So after being slammed with the first cruel wave and throwing out the anchor and trying things the recommended way, which were not the ones for me, I had to throw caution to the wind and hire the captain for my ship. Along the way, I wasn't surprised to find that my doctors were very supportive as they saw his results. More surprisingly was to find out how very little was known about these very conditions from which I suffered. RSDS has been documented from as far back as the days of the Civil War. I don't know about ANSD. My doctors learn willingly through my experiences. Even more surprising was the lack of diagnostic tools for RSDS and the cruel awakening that there was no cure but there was the hope of remission held out by Dr. Rhodes. With that being said, I would like to share part of my journal.

The pain of RSDS was unfathomable. There were guttural screams coming from the depths of my very core being from which I had never heard. The first doctor I sought treatment from was unable to provide a diagnosis, which resulted in a scathing letter from frustration. I received a diagnosis on my visit to a second doctor. Fortunately I was in the early stages and began receiving treatment promptly. I went the usual route of narcotics and ganglion blocks, which worked short term, but it became evident that

something else was going to be have to be done to ease my pain. I was broached with the possibility of a Spinal Cord Stimulator (SCS). I could not imagine a foreign object being implanted in my body. My psyche would not allow it. Here I was practically an invalid as a result of the RSDS with no place to go. I had clawed hands. My fingers were so swollen there came a day my wedding band had to be removed with bolt cutters as it was cutting off circulation to my finger. It was a traumatic event for me as it had never been off my finger. I tried to pretend my arms ended at my wrists and not my fingertips. They were hideous. A telephone was too heavy and difficult to manipulate. My bladder quit functioning for a few days. Bizarre things seemed to happen. As I lay on a table prior to one pain block I noticed my toes turning pink. Everyone in the room told me it was my runaway imagination. Was it? I wasn't blind but I kept silent. My sister was frantically searching for help. She came across a website which offered hope, www.paindefeat.com. To this day she considers this discovery her greatest feat in life. The only snag was it was a doctor in a totally different part of the country from where I lived. I could not imagine myself having an illness that could not be treated in my hometown in a way acceptable to me. But this doctor offered a treatment like no other. He did not use drugs of any sort, nor invasive treatment. He used electrode therapy. It was something that just had to be explored. With a family entourage we traveled to Corpus Christi, TX, full of hope. I must admit when we made the first attempt to find his clinic we drove right past it. The parking lot was so very small and the building was not all that inviting. We could not believe our hope lay beyond those doors. Nevertheless we persevered. Beyond those doors we met the most wonderful, gentle, caring people and, of course, Dr. Rhodes. We met other patients and their families and got to hear their stories. Right off the bat we knew we were in the right place. It was comforting to read all the letters written to Dr. Rhodes from former patients. They were proudly posted on a bulletin board for all to read. HIPAA was not around then and we had more freedom to mingle in the office. Our first trip was for two weeks and the subsequent one six months later was for three weeks. My hands were in pretty bad shape when we started treatment, but within about 1 ½ years of treatment the chronic pain of RSDS finally went into remission and my hands became fully functional. I was astonished.

Then I made a big mistake. At the time I went to remission I thought I was cured. I was ignorant. I didn't know then the things I do now about RSDS. More importantly, I didn't realize the relationship between the function of the ANSD and RSDS. If I had only asked more questions, I would never have put my home unit in its case, back in the closet, not to be used again. That is, until I came out of remission. But when your brain is so clouded with fog and you can no longer think like you used to because your memory is impaired, you don't realize your mistakes until after the fact. That is a hard and painful lesson.

I came out of remission from RSDS within a year. It crept up silently. One year after that, I was screaming in agony. I knew it was back. This time it had returned in my feet, ultimately affecting my ability to walk. I could no longer wear shoes. I made another mistake. I waited for a diagnosis instead of hopping on a plane straight to Corpus Christi, TX. I clung to false hope. I wanted to lay blame on my doctors but I only have myself to bear that burden. I lived in denial as I continued to deteriorate and in the long run only ended up hurting myself and my family even more. One day I received paperwork from one of my doctors to get a handicap parking tag. I went to the office of the county clerk, applied and received the tag. I hobbled out of the office and sat on the ground and cried. I didn't have it in me to walk to my car as my feet were in too much pain. I had not parked in a handicap spot, as I did not have the tag when I entered the office. My car seemed miles away when I walked out of the office. I finally drew on some inner strength to get to my car and screamed and cried all the way home. Any pride and guilt I may have had over applying for the tag very quickly evaporated.

I have had many problems. Let me give you a rundown of what I experienced: panic attacks, anxiety, prolonged adrenaline rushes, stress triggers, isolation, loneliness, foggy memory, mood swings, dry eyes, irritated corneas, facial flushes, inability to sweat, migraines, muscle spasms, weight fluctuations, nausea, joint pain, fatigue, insomnia, burning, numbness, tingling, skin discoloration in affected limbs, swelling, aching, stiffness, ringing ears, teeth grinding, dizziness, loose joints, weakened ligaments, diarrhea, constipation, irritable bowels, allergies, bone loss, subchondral cysts and an overwhelming burden of guilt. This list is in no particular order and I am sure there are more, but it gives one an idea of the magnitude of symptoms.

Coming out of remission and facing it was harder for me because, unlike the first go round, I knew what was in store for me and didn't want it to be real. If I went to Texas right off the bat it would be an admission I wasn't ready to make. It was easier to wait. Retrospectively, I keep kicking myself until I am black and blue all over. Wishing does not make it go away. Fear of travel gets you nowhere fast. One of my doctors recently told me, "Only you know your body. When RSDS hits, seek treatment immediately, especially if you have a doctor you know can help you." I admit to suppressing giggles as one of my doctors mumbles under his breath when writing references on my chart to ANSD. I know it causes him consternation. I have shared with another doctor: "Please listen to my words carefully in an office visit and if I ever give the hint of something seeming to be slightly askew, please call me on it so I can get help immediately." Another doctor is very adept at helping me find words when I am at a loss as to how to express my feelings. She encourages me to find my own way and get to Texas.

It has now been six years since I met Dr. Rhodes. RSDS is a very difficult condition to diagnose unless you are fortunate enough to run into a doctor who has seen it before. Dr. Rhodes uses a combination of several tests as his diagnostic tools. In the years I have been coming to see him, he has relocated his office to its third location, each time bigger. This lone ranger has gotten the RSDS to go into remission once, and we are currently working on trying to get it into remission again. I don't think I gave the home unit enough time to help with my ANSD. I was ignorant of so many things when I first started my ventures to Texas, probably because I was so sick. But now I am much wiser. I have learned through my own experience and research after the fact that RSDS does not go away, that it does go into remission. I still have to deal with ANSD. I now know how to listen very acutely to the warning signals in my body. I have learned the hard way that it is truly okay to question and even challenge your doctors when in your heart you just know something is just not quite right. RSDS and ANSD are not things to be taken lightly and they need to be tackled head on. You have to face your fear. Ignorance is not bliss, it will not make it go away, in fact it will only increase stress and make things much worse. It has taken trial and error, but I have figured out the most efficient and refined means of communicating my pain issues to Dr. Rhodes. I have learned to trace my hands and feet to better identify changing areas of pain and use a lot of verbiage on my pain grids to get the most efficient treatment protocol. I am still fascinated that sometimes I can see results within a day.

During my most recent trip, Dr. Rhodes developed a brand new treatment protocol just for me. I had him autograph it because he has helped me. Because of my ANSD, it is vital to my well-being that I do my therapy daily for the rest of my life to keep my body in sync. I am slowly coming out of a fog and maybe some day I will become the person I never knew I could be. I have learned which medications from which to steer totally clear as they only serve to increase pain and interfere with optimal performance of my personalized home unit. The remaining medications I am taking have been given a hard look and, with the assistance of my doctors, I am whittling down as many as I can. I am doing this with eyes wide open and admit it is a scary proposition for me, but in the long haul I cannot believe long term use of drugs is to my benefit. I am putting faith in Dr. Rhodes, as far as the full scope of the ANSD is concerned, just knowing in my heart my other doctors will be there to catch me if I fall and diagnose new symptoms as soon as they appear. I have learned the importance of opening up and sharing what I have learned with others. Dr. Rhodes has worked very hard to return some semblance of normalcy to my life when it all fell apart. I say normalcy and it is funny because I don't remember what that is like. I look forward to a different, more enriched life. I hate to imagine what my future would hold without Dr. Rhodes as an integral part of my health care team.

During the six years I have been dealing with RSDS and ANSD, I developed an adverse reaction to the electrodes used in the course of the therapy. I went to a skin allergist and found I was allergic to the acrylic in the adhesive of the electrodes. As a result I had to suspend therapy until I was able to find new ones that did not contain the allergen. I did this by contacting Dynatron, explained my dilemma and was told by them that there were hypoallergenic electrodes available and where to get them. For anyone in need, I use PALS Neurostimulation Electrodes, Reusable, Self-Adhering; Quadrastim; 1.25" (3CM) Round; Quantity 8 per Package; AXELGAARD MANUFACTURING CO., LTD.; Headquarters: Fallbrook, CA 92028 USA; Europe:DK-8520 Lystrup, Denmark; E-Mail: support@axelgaard.com. You can contact Dynatron directly to find a distributor near you.

I had some rare opportunities with Dr. Rhodes. In the latter months of 2004 I had the privilege of being one of the first, if not the first, patients to be included in the Beta testing phase of one of his newest pieces of equipment, which now has a patent pending. Ironically enough, in January of 2006 I was in his clinic being tested by said piece of equipment and was observed by his patent attorney. I was so excited to be involved in that process. In mid-2006 I was in his office when he found out good news about his work with diabetes and how I could look forward to his publication sometime in the near term. It could open so many doors for him. I feel he is just on the brink of something big. Reflex Sympathetic Dystrophy Syndrome was just a starting point for Dr. Rhodes. He is a fascinating man who is so passionate about easing the pain of others. He has never stopped studying the human body and its biochemistry. I love to listen to his stories of success, discovery and hopes for the future. He does not like to fail. Sometimes I find him intimidating just because of his size but once I get past that he is a very easy person with whom to share pain. I enjoy chance meetings with other patients and hearing their firsthand stories. An added benefit is that Corpus Christi, TX is full of wonderful people and it affords a climate conducive to healing.

Dr. Rhodes is on the brink of getting his technology launched into and accepted by the medical community at large. I can feel it in my heart. There are so many people suffering and at the end of the line and he can offer hope. Please visit his website at www.paindefeat.com. You could be enlightened as I was and find your captain. Perhaps after reading this Dr. Rhodes will be your first choice to banish your pain and not your last.

There are some things I have not included as I wish to keep them private, others have been purged from my memory as they were too painful to retain. Nevertheless, the pain inflicted on my mind, body and spirit has been horrendous. Unless you have walked a mile in my shoes you can only imagine what it is like and even doing that will not get you close. I have learned life lessons and the value of family and friends. I have learned to live for the moment and not to worry about tomorrow. It is a much more peaceful existence. Maintaining a positive attitude is such a crucial part of the healing process as well as knowing that you will stumble along the way, reach plateaus, improve and hopefully reach your goal. Perseverance is the key.

I would be remiss if I did not mention one more thing: Surgery. Said topic of any kind is out of the question for me unless it becomes a life threatening situation due to the risk of the spread of RSDS. Contrary to popular belief, even if it is in a non-limb affected area of the body, RSDS can flair anywhere. I have learned this not only from Dr. Rhodes but in speaking with other patients in his clinic. I was faced with the possibility of surgery in my hand in recent years. In fact it was even scheduled. Something was nagging at the back of my mind to seek a second opinion. I went to my neurologist and sought his counsel. He advised against it. I went home, gave the discussion some thought and cancelled the surgery. At the time I did not realize what a life altering decision that was and I suspect he did not realize the magnitude of it either. I will be eternally grateful.

I would like to thank my family and team of physicians who have staunchly stood by my side and held my hand through thick and thin and offered a willingness to learn through my experiences. It is funny; some families are torn apart by the horrors of this condition, but in my case, my family has been drawn closer together. I consider myself very fortunate. My Mother has been my traveling companion, caregiver and confidante. My Father has been my chauffeur on countless occasions, spent endless hours in waiting rooms watching paint dry and learned the hard way that bad things don't go away. We have had good moments sharing a cup of coffee and drawing on napkins. My sister and brothers will drop anything, anytime to come running to my assistance. My special girlfriend willingly spends countless hours on the phone with me dealing with all of my mood swings about living life in a black hole wondering if I would ever again see the light of day. I have more close relatives and friends who have stuck by me and I have somehow recruited others along the way as I journey toward my future.

A special thank you to Dr. Rhodes for accepting the enormous challenge presented to him by Maria in 1992, for had he not, he would not be in the position he is to help me today. I was once asked over two decades ago: "What is the purpose of your life?" Maybe I have found it. Maybe sharing a glimpse into my journal and talking about my experiences is it. Thank you for taking the time to read my words. If they reach just one person then I know they were worth sharing.

Tamara, USA

Readers' Comments:

"…. Touching, heart wrenching story of a woman who came back from the depths…Must read. You'll come away inspired to carry on with your own battles." – Julia Tirpak

"….This story gives the old cliché, "Walk a mile in my shoes" a whole NEW meaning."...Libby Turner

"…..This is terribly painful to read when you love the person who wrote it. I simply can't believe she endured these things to this extent and I didn't know it. I've been stumped for several weeks to put my reaction in writing. May the worst be over for her and may she have helped the doctors and other patients in her expression of her reality." Godmother, Elaine Baer

~~~~~~

Jennifer

I'm a pediatrician. I hadn't worked full time in more than a year. Finally,
I felt so bad I had to give up my practice completely. The fatigue, pain,
chest tightness, shortness of breath, poor memory--I feared I might make
a medical error with disastrous consequences. My life was falling apart.

I had been tired since age fifteen after a bout with an illness that put me in bed for two months. It was diagnosed as rheumatic fever. It wasn't until I was in medical school that I realized I had less endurance than other people. In my third year of training I realized that in addition to the fatigue, I had been hurting all over for some time. I just assumed everybody felt that way. Then I developed intense hip pain. I needed to lose weight, so I exercised. That helped with the fatigue but made the hip pain worse. As a doctoral student, I learned the clinical symptoms of fibromyalgia and figured out that must be my problem. However, I was told that fibromyalgia was all in the head.

After medical school I married, gave birth to two children, and set up my medical practice. During the second pregnancy, I began to forget things. And I always felt really, really tired. I began to experience vision changes, shortness of breath, and worsening of an over active bladder condition. I suffered from depression. I struggled along through the years, pushing myself every day in order to keep my life on track. I was often cranky, so much so that I ran off two husbands. I still thought everybody felt as I did, that everyone lived in misery but just didn't talk about it.

When I developed hives, I put myself on steroids and exercised. I felt somewhat better but was still depressed, tired, and in pain. I continued to deteriorate. I couldn't sleep, I was often nauseated, felt cold, and was irritable all the time.

That's when I began to realize how bad my memory had become. I was forgetting important information. I had an associate in my pediatric practice and managed for a while to keep my clinic going by relying on my colleague. But I kept getting worse. So, I cut back on my hours, took fewer patients, and tried to lower my stress level. I am a very wound up type of person and know now that's a contributing factor for pain syndromes.

However, I continued to get worse. My hair started falling out, I often couldn't get out of bed, but my blood tests showed nothing wrong. What I did have was a specific physical reaction to the fibromyalgia trigger points. So, in spite of what I had been told in medical school about that condition being "in the head," I knew I had it. But no one seemed to know how to treat it.

Finally, when I hadn't worked full time in more than a year and continued to get worse, I realized I had to give up my practice completely. The fatigue, pain, chest tightness, shortness of breath, poor memory--I feared I might make a medical error with disastrous consequences. My life was falling apart.

That was when I learned about Dr. Rhodes. I decided to give him a try. I came into his clinic with a pain level of between seven and eight. Plus I still had all the other symptoms. After two and a half weeks of treatments, I was better than I had felt in three or four years. After the fifteenth day of treatment, I left the Dr. Rhodes' clinic with a pain level of between zero and two. With further treatments, I continued to improve. My morale was higher, my fatigue was lifting, my mood was more cheerful, and my memory was improving.

As I learned more about the underlying problem in my body that had triggered my condition, I realized I was predisposed to fibromyalgia. Tightly wound people like me produce too much norepinephrine. When that substance, which should last only twenty seconds in the body, hangs around for twenty minutes instead, it makes the individual hypertensive and eats away at the nerves. It can produce a wide variety of symptoms that often baffle doctors when they can find no specific illness present.

I am so grateful that Dr. Rhodes has developed a treatment for people like me. I have come a long way. I have my life back, I am engaged to a wonderful man with whom I am not cranky, my memory is back to normal, my vision is stable, I don't hurt, I am optimistic, I am energetic. In other words, I feel normal for the first time since I was fifteen years old. I finally have a life. What a gift.

~~~~~

Melissa and Alberto Belalcazar

Corpus Christi, Texas

Three out-of-state women who came into our medical clinic for cosmetic procedures said, "You've got a doctor in this town who is doing miraculous things." It's hard to believe that a doctor could be doing such wonderful work in a clinic right around the corner from ours, and I didn't even know about him.

Melissa:

My husband and I have been married for three years. He is a general surgeon, who at my encouragement, has expanded into cosmetic surgery. A while back three separate women from out of state came to our clinic at different times for Botox® treatments while in town for another reason. The first one came from Hawaii. The second one was from Ohio. I don't recall where the third one lived, but they had all come into town for the same initial reason. And each one said basically the same thing to me, "I came all this way from home to be treated for pain. You've got a doctor in this town who is doing miraculous things."

After the first lady, I was skeptical. The second one tweaked my interest. But when the third one showed up, I said to myself, "That's it. I'm calling him. It must be a sign."

I've lived with pain most of my life. My mother said that as I child, I would hit my head on the wall and scream. As far back as I can remember, I've had migraines. They would strike every two weeks and last three to four days. Then fifteen years ago at my 30th birthday party, I kept doing the limbo over and over again. That set up chronic pain in my back. At age 35, I had a sledding accident that broke my tailbone. My pain level skyrocketed. There were days I would pray to God to take me with him. This went on for ten years. I went to chiropractors, had massages, and took very expensive medication for my back and the migraines. At one time, I was up to eight aspirin a day, which caused me to get stomach ulcers. I had to stop taking them. I was in agony.

All that kept me going was the example of my nephew, Marco. He died at fourteen from bone cancer. That is an extremely painful condition. He had fifteen surgeries in five years. He didn't complain even though he suffered terribly. The cancer eventually went to his brain, and even with his terrible headaches, he would endure the pain. I thought, here I was hurting terribly, and he suffered more. He taught me how to be brave about suffering. If he could cope with it, I could, too.

When I met my husband, I lived in constant pain. I tried hard not to show it. After we married, I'd wake up most mornings in so much pain that when he would lean over to hug me, I couldn't bear it. I would tell him not to touch me. My body ached too much. I tried hard to keep my distress to myself, but I was always somewhat withdrawn.

So when those female patients came one by one to our clinic and raved about our local miracle doctor I went to see him because I was desperate for some sort of relief.

After two months of treatment, my pain level has dropped from a ten to a one and even a zero most of the time. I haven't felt like this since I was twenty, and I'm forty-five. It's wonderful to feel normal. I had forgotten what it was like to walk around with no pain.

My husband was so surprised when I began waking up happy. He was so intrigued with what Dr. Rhodes had done for me that he became a believer and is also being treated by Dr. Rhodes.

My eighty-two-year-old dad has Parkinson's and my mother suffers from headaches due to an inoperable brain tumor, diabetes, and body aches. I convinced them to see Dr. Rhodes. My dad's speech is better, and he doesn't shuffle when he walks the way he did before. My mother's shoulder pain is gone and her headaches improved. Now my sister, who was once skeptical, is also being treated for her back pain and headaches. Since RSD-type conditions are inherited, my whole family can benefit from Dr. Rhodes' treatments.

My genetic makeup will require that I use the machine for the rest of my life. But that's okay because I feel so good. I feel blessed to have learned about Dr. Rhodes. It's hard to believe that a doctor could be doing such wonderful work in a clinic right around the corner from ours, and I didn't even know about him until patients from out of state informed me. Everyone needs to know about him. He is wonderful. I just love him.

Alberto Belalcazar, M.D.

I went to Dr. Rhodes after I saw what he did for my wife, Melissa. I was astonished at how he transformed her life. I had to see it to believe it.

I had chronic constipation and high blood pressure. And there was another matter I wanted to check out. So I thought I'd give Dr. Rhodes a try. He said he could help me. He said we are like dogs. We are supposed to eat, then go to the bathroom, then eat and go to the bathroom. Well, I didn't follow that pattern. And it was a problem. After three weeks of treatment, my constipation is history.

Dr. Rhodes fixes one problem at a time, so next he tackled my high blood pressure. I am still on medication, but my pressure is dropping. While waiting to get to the third problem, I did some research on VIP. I learned that it plays a part in a great number of conditions. For one, it decreases high blood pressure, a positive effect which I was already experiencing from the treatments. The body also produces it in the genitals, where it helps with functions in that part of the anatomy.

Now I was learning something very interesting. With Dr. Rhodes' machine, I can look forward to a Viagra-like effect. He said it's worked on other patients. And after what I've seen with how he's transformed Melissa, I believe he knows what he's talking about. Am I ever glad those young ladies from out of state came into our clinic.

~~~~~

Maddie

Medical discoveries sometimes are made by a lone individual who goes where others have not yet gone. And that person leads the way for everybody else. Dr. Rhodes is such an individual.

Kindy, Maddie's mother:

If only we could clone Dr. Rhodes! What he has done for Maddie is a miracle. I cannot say enough about him. He needs to train medical personnel all over the country to treat people with RSD, because he is the one with the answers. One doctor who treated Maddie offered us no hope. He said, "There's no one who understands this disease—-no one who can do anything about it." We know now that is not true.

Doctors do the best they can to treat this kind of pain, but Dr. Rhodes has developed the only method that works. We know. We searched the Internet, went to doctor after doctor, had all kinds of therapies for Maddie, but nothing helped. She only got worse. At age 12 her life was turned into a never-ending nightmare.

It began with shooting, stabbing pains in Maddie's feet, and then began shooting up her legs. Of course, we now know that it was the beginning of RSD, but was diagnosed at the time as falling arches. We were told to purchase shoe inserts, give her motrin for the pain, and follow up in six months. We went back before the six month mark, where the doctor decided surgery was needed to create arches in her feet.

I had no idea then that the operation was the worst thing anyone could have done to my daughter. I was completely unaware of RSD and its characteristics. If only we had had that knowledge, we could have avoided so much pain and confusion.

In the recovery room after my daughter's initial surgery, she woke to extreme pain. She was sobbing and screaming. There was confusion with the staff, thinking it may have been spasms in her feet. She was given high doses of valium to calm her. I seemed to be the only one who believed there was something more than muscle spasms. Everyone seemed to think she was perhaps dramatizing.

Both feet were to remain in the casts, with zero weight bearing for the first month. Within two days of bringing Maddie home, we returned to the hospital. When the doctor saw Maddie, he said he believed she had RSD. An appointment was scheduled later that afternoon with a pain clinic, where they could not confirm her condition due to her heavy sedation and inability to look at her casted feet. I held my daughter's head in my arms for the first three weeks. She took pain medications, but the agony was so intense, she would lose consciousness.

She then went to physical therapy, but everything they did for her only made matters worse. She would cry, "What's wrong with me?" Everyone, including her physical therapist, did not understand and thought she might be faking. I was the only person throughout this whole ordeal who really believed something was desperately wrong with my daughter.

To make matters worse, Maddie underwent a second surgery six months after her first, by a different doctor. He wanted to explore inside her feet to look for any impingements, or errors from the first operation. He found nothing wrong. Of course, the second operation was also a major mistake. The change in her life was enormous. Her memory was poor. She became isolated from friends and even family, who at times doubted her pain. They thought she just wanted attention.

As a divorced mother who was our sole support, I was working and would have to leave her alone at home during the day. There was no way she could attend school. She experienced daily panic attacks and would call me in tears. I used all my sick and vacation time attending to her needs. Her older brother also suffered from seeing his sister in such bad shape. Our lives were crumbling around our feet. I cannot count the nights I spent on my knees in tears and prayer.

I called pain doctors frantically searching for some clue about my daughter's condition and found a wonderful doctor, who was the first to give us any hope. He knew immediately what she had and made the RSD diagnosis. She was placed on narcotics and given three spinal blocks. Unfortunately, her relief lasted only minutes.

Eventually, we found another doctor that we thought was a medical pioneer. Maddie had a knee block, then a pic-line (which is an IV threaded directly into the heart). Anesthesia ran through this IV 24/7 for two solid weeks. The pain, however, remained and sometimes increased. We tried everything imaginable, but Maddie ended up just living on a number of narcotics.

I could not believe the amount of pain my daughter continued to suffer. We spent days with her crying and screaming and sometimes fainting, with no relief in sight.

After a year of this heartbreak, I found Dr. Rhodes on the Internet. I took the printed information from his website to our pain management doctor's office, but he told us there was nothing anyone could do, that he himself was our best bet.

After another painful year, Dr. Rhodes' name found us again. I believe divine intervention brought us back to his website. I just knew this was where we needed to be. He seemed to be a cross between a mad scientist and a genius, just the kind of person who would develop something revolutionary.

Yet in spite of all the wonderful testimonials on Dr. Rhodes' website, I could not help but feel a bit skeptical. But when I reflected on what Maddie's chronic pain had done to all of us, I knew I had to take a chance on the one doctor who said he could help. I was frantic after two years of watching my daughter's unimaginable suffering.

Before RSD, Maddie had played tennis and won races at school. She had received prizes for her accomplishments. She was in gifted classes and excelled in everything she did.

As for Dr. Rhodes, what other choice did I have? He was our only hope. So I refinanced my house, asked for a two--week leave from my job (without pay), and took my daughter to Texas. To add to the trauma, Maddie had to withdraw from the narcotics so that the treatment would work successfully. She fainted many times, and once, ended up in the emergency room. Our two weeks turned into seven and my employer let me go. We came home, only to return to Texas for two more months.

There is no question we had doubts about the treatment the first few weeks. Progress seemed so slow. What kept us going was Dr. Rhodes' encouragement and talking to other patients who were recovering. When Maddie arrived at the clinic, her pain level was a 9/10. After two and a half months, she's off of all narcotics, and her pain is consistently at 5/6. That is remarkable since she has many obstacles to overcome. First, her feet were so sensitive that she could not tolerate the electrodes on them for seven weeks. The surgery incisions are also in the exact area the electrodes are to be placed. Therefore, the progress was much slower, because they had to be placed on her legs. The scar tissue also blocks the electrical stimulation from its full intensity, so that too is a detriment. Also, she is female and fifteen years old (which is the most difficult age group to treat). In spite of these problems, Maddie feels better than she has in two years.

Maddie and I are so encouraged. We came to the right place. We've seen others get well, and we know Maddie will make it, too. She's already come so far. And we have one incredibly wonderful man to thank for that, Dr. Rhodes.

If only we had known the signs of the disease, Maddie would have been spared so much pain. Her life would not have been derailed for those years. We would have saved so much money.

We can't undo the past, but we can pass on what we know to others. By doing so, maybe we can spare them the fruitless journey through failed therapies and unrelenting pain. Anyone in chronic pain who cannot get relief from non-invasive therapies should check out Dr. Rhodes before submitting to surgery, narcotics, and other procedures that can do more damage than good.

Remember, medical discoveries sometimes are made by a lone individual who goes where others have not yet gone. And that person leads the way for everybody else. Dr. Rhodes is such an individual.

~~~~~

Jack

When I first went to Dr. Rhodes, I needed wheel chair assistance to travel. I could walk only a hundred yards. Now I can accomplish my "honey-do list" around the house, perform light-weight floor exercises, and I'm rebuilding my body at age 78.

I had polio at age 21. I don't know if it contributed to my later arthritic back pain. But it certainly didn't hold me back when I was younger. Most of my life I was extremely active. I scuba dived, swam, skied, hiked, climbed mountains, and engaged in other strenuous activities for recreation. In my mid-fifties, I developed periodic episodes of back pain that would resolve. I retired at age fifty-seven and spent two years seeing the world, devoting even more time to my favorite sports. I came back to the U.S. and stayed active. I had no serious physical problems at that time.

Then I began having trouble with my left hip, which doctors discovered had deteriorated from arthritis. (Doctors in all medical specialties refer to bone deterioration, honeycombing, and collapse as arthritis. The pain results from deformed bones or bulging disks pressing on nerves.) I had a total hip replacement. Then I had periodic onsets of back pain. While arthritis had been busy deteriorating my hip, it had also deteriorated bones in my back. I took medications for the pain.

One day, seven or eight years after the operation, I developed such excruciating pain in my right hip and lower back that I was immobilized. I literally could not move. I took more than 1,400 mg. of ibuprofen before I got enough relief so I could move and get out of bed. I faced this every day for a couple of months before an orthopedic surgeon talked about back surgery.

Before I could make a decision, I found myself in worse shape than I thought. I had to have an aortic heart valve replaced and triple bypass surgery. Although I recovered from the surgery, I was pretty much immobilized for three months, during which time I was, naturally, very inactive. So, my back pain lessened.

When I became more mobile and more active, my back pain started again. I had a cervical fusion in the spine between C2 and C3, with a satisfactory outcome. Then the debilitating pain occurred in my lower back with the same diagnosis of destructive arthritis. The doctors advised against more surgery and suggested drug therapy, which I started. I was able to be mobile for about five hours a day. But my mobility was limited. I couldn't even take walks and was headed for a life of immobility and pain.

Then I learned about Dr. Rhodes and decided to see him. After two months of treatment, I was off all drugs. My pain level started to decrease. I was more mobile but not yet active. After ten months of regular treatment, mostly at home, my pain level varies from zero to two. I am very mobile now and travel without a wheel chair. You see, when I first went to Dr. Rhodes, I had to travel as a handicapped person, needing wheel chair assistance. I could walk a hundred yards or so. No further. That was then.

Today, I can handle the "honey-do" list for house maintenance. I can perform light-weight floor exercises and stretching. I am trying to recover my muscle strength. In trying to rebuild my body at age 78, I also maintain a healthful lifestyle and attitude.

For me, drugs were absolutely not an acceptable treatment or way of life. I would have had to take them forever. Dr. Rhodes' methodology appeared to me to treat the cause of the problem, not just the symptoms. It was worth trying. And I'm grateful for the results. I am so much better now without the drugs and with Dr. Rhodes' machine than I ever was or could have been with drugs and without the machine.

~~~~~~

"I have lived with chronic pain from more than thirty years, and nothing has given me more relief than Dr. Rhodes' treatments. His machine even cleaned out the excess protein in my kidneys."

Jose

PART THREE—CLINICAL AND SCHOLARLY RESEARCH

BY: DR. DONALD RHODES

The following is for those interested in information of a more technical nature.

RSDS/CRPS AND FIBROMYALGIA AND THE BASIC CAUSES OF PAIN

Many diseases (including RSDS/CRPS and Fibromyalgia) trace their origin to a breakdown in the stress response system of the body. The human stress response system (primarily the sympathetic nervous system which is the more active portion of the autonomic nervous system) is designed to protect the body from real or perceived threats. This is the fight, flight, or fright system. This system is designed to have a physical reaction to a short-term stress. When a threat is perceived, the body reacts with a "mass discharge" of norepinephrine from the adrenal glands. Norepinephrine helps to protect the body by changing the allocation of circulation and by changing carbohydrate metabolism. This is a protective mechanism that is designed to change the body's focus for approximately 20 seconds to survive a threat. Norepinephrine increases the flow of blood to the large muscles at the expense of the digestive system, small muscles, nerves, bone, and skin. Not only is the heart rate increased but also the pulse volume of the heart is increased by as much as 50%. Norepinephrine causes the release of insulin and the breakdown of glycogen, the "storehouse of sugar." The insulin allows the large muscles to utilize the blood sugar more efficiently.

This stress response system was well adapted for human life 50,000 years ago when stresses were of short duration and were handled with a physical response. However, in the modern era, stress is rarely short-term and usually cannot be dealt with by a physical response. Those areas of the body which are denied adequate circulation by the stress response system have no problem tolerating insufficient circulation of 20 seconds. However, these areas cannot tolerate continued insufficient circulation for extended periods of time. Many different diseases are caused by insufficient circulation to the digestive system, small muscles, nerves, bone, and skin. In essence, this is a stone-age physiology in a space age world.

Under normal circumstances, the circulation to a given part of the body is determined by demand, since supply is adequate. The autonomic nervous system and various neuropeptides control the flow of blood. VIP (vasoactive intestinal polypeptide) increases the blood flow to the intestinal tract. The flow of blood to the skin, nerves, bone, and small muscles is increased by CGRP (calcitonin gene-related peptide). This increased flow is decreased by neurons releasing substance P, which causes the mast cells to release a proteolytic enzyme, which destroys CGRP. In a "normal" human, there is a balance between norepinephrine/substance P, decreasing the blood flow to these various tissues and organs, while CGRP and VIP increase the blood flow.

Norepinephrine is destroyed on a system-wide basis by catecholamine-O-methyl transferase (COMT). The amount of COMT made by an individual's body is determined by their genetic makeup. There are two COMT alleles, valine and methionine. The valine COMT produces a normal amount of COMT. The methionine COMT produces much less COMT. The COMT genes follow Mendelian genetics. Dr. Jan Zubieta performed the pioneer investigation into the action of these genes. He found that persons with a low/low COMT (met/met) or low/high COMT (met/val) genes were less able to tolerate pain than persons with a high/high COMT (val/val) gene. PET scans showed that this occurred because the people with met/met COMT or met/val COMT made less beta-endorphins. In addition, the decreased COMT levels allowed the norepinephrine produced by the sympathetic nervous system to last much longer in their bodies. He found that approximately 25% of the people in the United States have met/met and val/val COMT genes, while 50% of the people have met/val COMT genes. When he studied those patients complaining of severe pain, he found that their genetic makeup was usually met/met COMT or sometimes met/val but only extremely rarely val/val COMT.

When norepinephrine is released from the adrenal glands in patients with val/val COMT, it remains very active for approximately 20 seconds and semi-active for several minutes. However, in patients with met/met or met/val COMT, the norepinephrine remains very active for 2 or 3 minutes and semi-active for at least 6 minutes. In addition, he found that people who had val/val COMT were able to tolerate much more pain than people who had met/met COMT. PET scans confirmed that this was probably due to the normal production of beta-endorphins in response to pain. It has been found that the bulk of patients with diseases such as Fibromyalgia and RSDS and other forms of severe chronic pain usually are patients with less than normal levels of COMT.

The increased duration of the action of norepinephrine causes ischemia in the skin, nerves, bone, small muscles, and in the intestinal tract. This ischemia causes pain, which liberates substance P, the chemical transmitter of pain. Substance P causes the mast cells to produce a proteolytic enzyme that destroys CGRP, which results in increased ischemia and, therefore, increased pain. This becomes a circle of continually worsening ischemia and pain.

In addition, the longer duration of norepinephrine causes a marked increased liberation of insulin. This places an increase stress on the beta cells in the Islets of Langerhans, which produce the insulin. This requires an increased supply of oxygen at the very time that circulation to this area is being decreased. Of the entire body, the three areas which are the most sensitive to oxygen deprivation are the central nervous system, the peripheral nervous system, and the Islets of Langerhans. This decreased oxygen causes increased reactive oxygen species, which cause mutations in the mitochondrial chromosomes and interferes in the production of ATP and, therefore, decreases the production of insulin.

There is an increasing body of scientific evidence that ischemia in tissues is the etiology of disease. Ischemia causes a buildup of reactive oxygen species (ROS) and changes the local pH of tissues. Since the circulation is decreased, there is an accumulation of CO2. The CO2 combines with water to become carbonic acid. As the pH decreases, various deleterious changes occur.

The decreased oxygen has been shown to be responsible for an increase in tumor necrosis factor alpha, vascular endothelium growth factor, and various cytokines. These substances are responsible for such varied disease such as Rheumatoid arthritis, endometriosis, and diabetic retinopathy, as well as worsening RSDS/CRPS and Fibromyalgia. TNF alpha has been shown to increase insulin resistance throughout the body, which makes the symptoms of RSDS much worse. Increased insulin resistance causes increased blood glucose. It has been demonstrated that when the blood glucose is higher than 130 mg%, COMT is deactivated. This allows for increased norepinephrine activity, which exacerbates the signs and symptoms of RSDS.

Many of these diseases affect women more that men. This is probably because men have a better oxygen supply to the periphery of their bodies. In general, men have higher blood pressures than women. Men have more muscle than women and, therefore, have more myoglobin, which holds oxygen in the muscles. In addition, men have more hemoglobin than women. Women have 12 to 14 mg% hemoglobin in their blood while men have 14 to 17 mg%. Diseases such as RSDS, Fibromyalgia, and Chronic Fatigue Syndrome affect mostly women.

In bone, the decreased oxygen and decreased pH are responsible for a breakdown of the bone matrix. Bone is a matrix of hydroxyapatite and collagen held together with copper in a matrix maintained by a Piezo electric current. The stress side of the bone has a negative charge and the compressive side of the bone has a positive charge. Osteoblasts, which are responsible for the building of bone, go primarily to the negative (stress) side of the bone. Osteoclasts, which are responsible for the remodeling of bone, go primarily to the positive (compressive) side of the bone. This loss of bone shows up first in the areas of increased oxygen use. Therefore, it is seen as subchondral cystic degeneration beneath cartilage or where there is an attachment of muscles, tendons, or ligaments. With time this becomes more generalized and is seen as osteopenia and, eventually, as osteoporosis. If these subchondral cysts are in a line, a pathological fracture may occur.

The cartilage has no intrinsic circulation and derives all of its nutrients and rids itself of its waste products into the underlying bone. However, if the underlying bone no longer exists and is now a subchondral cyst, the cartilage begins to degenerate. This is seen as degenerative joint disease or arthritis. These bone cysts increase in size with low barometric pressure, which is why RSDS patients' pain is many times radically increased with rainy weather.

The skin, being deprived of adequate circulation, begins to break down and is seen as nonhealing ulcerations, nonpruritic lichenification, and occasionally cellulitis.

Cells in the small muscles, being deprived of adequate circulation, begin having small areas of cell death. This is seen clinically as tremors, fasciculations, or in diseases such as RSDS or Fibromyalgia.

The nerves in the central nervous system and peripheral nervous system, being deprived of adequate circulation, begin to degenerate. Myelin is extremely sensitive to oxygen deprivation. As the myelin degenerates, the nerves transmit with less than normal stimulation (hyperesthetic). With continued hypoxia, the nerves only transmit with more than normal stimulation (hypoesthetic). Eventually, with continued hypoxia, the nerves will not transmit (anesthetic). Saltatory conduction suffers and nerve conduction velocity is decreased. Since nerve conduction velocity only tests the A-beta fibers and only show decreased nerve conduction, these studies are useless in early RSDS. The hyperesthetic nerves will result in a normal reading. Many times, this causes intense frustration on the part of the RSDS patient since they would be told that the NCV testing did not indicate malfunctioning nerves.

One of the aspects of this situation, which is usually overlooked, is that the nerves are the source of the neuropeptides, which counteract norepinephrine. Nerves throughout the body create CGRP and VIP. However, when the nerves do not receive adequate oxygen to function normally, they do not make adequate amounts of the neuropeptides.

Norepinephrine is destroyed by COMT. However, patients with chronic pain do not have adequate COMT. The only other substance within the body which is known to destroy norepinephrine is melatonin. The problem is that melatonin is produced by the pineal gland in the presence of adequate VIP and cAMP (cyclic adenosine monophosphate), which are produced by nerves. Since these nerves are not receiving adequate oxygen, the VIP and cAMP are not being produced in adequate amounts to create the melatonin to destroy the norepinephrine. In addition, melatonin is produced after 4 P.M. due to the body's circadian rhythm. At approximately 4 P.M., the body's blood cortisol level, blood beta-endorphin level, and blood pressure decrease. At approximately 4 A.M., these levels increase. This helps explain why chronic pain patients have insomnia and increased pain in the evening and are able to sleep better during the daytime.

This inability to produce adequate VIP and cAMP creates diseases as diverse as migraine headaches, Irritable Bowel Syndrome, and asthma. Many RSDS patients suffer from these diseases without realizing that they are all connected.

Migraine headaches occur due to a lack of glycogen. The brain utilizes glycogen for energy. Glycogen requires one half of the oxygen to metabolize as does blood glucose. However, the body requires VIP to create glycogen. Therefore, if there is not adequate VIP the brain is forced to utilize blood glucose, which requires more oxygen to metabolize, at a time of decreased oxygen supply.

Irritable Bowel Syndrome occurs when there is insufficient VIP in the intestinal tract. This causes hypoxia in these tissues.

Medical literature has shown that asthmatic patients have markedly decreased VIP producing nerves in their lungs.

VIP and beta-endorphins determine the immune system function of the body. These neuropeptides are diminished in RSDS and Fibromyalgia, which causes RSDS patients to be prone to illness such as the flu and slow to recover from these illnesses.

Many RSDS and Fibromyalgia patients are also diagnosed as having Raynaud's Disease or Phenomenon. Raynaud's Disease/Phenomenon is caused by a lack of CGRP producing neurons in the skin. RSDS and Fibromyalgia have the same pathology.

Normally, dynorphins, beta-endorphins, and enkephalins inhibit the release of norepinephrine. However, in patients with insufficient amounts of COMT, the production of these neuropeptides is diminished. As was seen earlier, these are patients who experience significant amounts of pain. If this type of patient is seen by a physician and complains of moderate to severe pain, the physician is liable to write a prescription for a morphine derivative mediation. These medicines may dull the painful sensations; however, they actually make the chronic pain syndrome worse. This is also true of the nonnarcotic drugs, which function in the body as a narcotic, such as Ultram. All of these medicines decrease the production of dynorphins, enkephalins, and beta-endorphins. Studies have shown that narcotics increase the release of norepinephrine 200 to 300%. Even worse reactions have been found if the patient misses a dosage of the narcotic or intentionally tries to diminish the amount of daily intake of the narcotic. It has been found that reduction of the daily intake of narcotics doubles the output of norepinephrine.

Patients in our clinic are never prescribed narcotics, except during the course of reduction of their previously prescribed narcotics. When a patient arrives at our clinic utilizing narcotics or other deleterious medications, they are prescribed a slow reduction to prevent exacerbations of the RSDS, due to the withdrawal of the medications. It is necessary for the patient to be off all narcotics to be able to return to a normal pain-free life.

I am the inventor and patent holder of the methodology of what is in the FDA approved physical therapy system known as the Dynatronic STS. This system involves two simultaneous, separate interferential treatments. STS treatments are designed to normalize the abnormal autonomic nervous system. The current working hypothesis is that the STS treatments are effective due to a combination of the following aspects of the treatments: low frequency electrical current passing through long sections of nerves; electrode pad placement (including acupuncture and reflexology points); production of cyclic adenosine monophosphate; the choice of the peripheral nerves being stimulated so that there is a cross-over effect in the Central Nervous System; leakage of action potentials from the nerves being stimulated into nerves entering the sympathetic ganglia; the quadrilateral location of stimulation; creation of action potentials through sympathetic nerve fibers, in the peripheral nerves being stimulated; creation of action potentials in peripheral nerves being stimulated; activation of the sodium pump, in the nerves being stimulated; production of ACTH; production of dynorphins, enkephalins or beta-endorphins; creation of action potentials in sympathetic fibers within the peripheral nerves being stimulated, which enter the sympathetic ganglia directly; analgesia causing a reduction in the production of substance P; and/or the production of circulation altering neuropeptides such as vasoactive intestinal polypeptide(VIP) and calcitonin gene-related peptide (CGRP).

There are literally thousands of different combinations of beat frequencies and electrode pad placement protocols, which are utilized for our patients. The choice of electrode placement and beat frequency is unique to each patient and changes as often as necessary. Many times, these are changed on a daily basis to respond to the ever-changing RSDS symptoms.

An indication of autonomic nervous system (ANS) dysfunction is an alteration of the heart rate variability (HRV). HRV not only shows the relative control of the heart by the sympathetic and parasympathetic nervous system but also shows the heart rate variability compared to normal for that type of patient (based upon sex, age, marital status, etc.). Multiple HRV testing has shown that even the first STS treatment decreases the dominance of the sympathetic nervous system control of the heart and partially or fully normalizes the variability in the heart rate.

An indication of ANS dysfunction is nonhealing skin ulcerations. It has been found that STS treatments cause nonhealing ulcerations to granulate and heal. This has been documented with dated photographs.

Another indication of ANS dysfunction is the skin temperature and the skin temperature differential between the left and the right side of the body. Decreased skin temperature is an indication of decreased circulation into the skin vascular bed. The skin vascular bed circulation is increased by CGRP. In the absence of increased ambient temperature, if the skin temperature is increased, that is caused by an increased liberation of CGRP. Skin temperatures are taken from the lower and upper body. The palmar surface of the thumb should be approximately 91 degrees Fahrenheit. The plantar aspect of the big toe (hallux) should be approximately 83 degrees Fahrenheit. If there is a greater than a one-degree difference between the right and left sides and/or there is a lower or higher temperature of the fingers or toes, it indicates an ANS dysfunction. In the Peripheral Neuropathy study by Dr. Guido (published in the American Journal of Pain), it was shown that STS treatments normalize the actual skin temperature and also decrease the side-to-side variance of skin temperatures. That study also demonstrated that STS treatments radically increase the time and quality of sleep in chronic pain patients, indicating an increased production of melatonin. Medical literature has been demonstrated in multiple studies that a decreased endoneurial circulation causes decreased nerve conduction velocities (NCV). It has also been demonstrated that increased CGRP results in increased endoneurial circulation and normalization of decreased nerve conduction velocities. In the Guido study, 59% of the patients who had pre study and post study

NCV had nerve conduction improvement. This indicated that adequate CGRP was produced by the STS treatments.

Routinely in our office, it has been found that, utilizing STS treatments, we are able to normalize ANS dysfunction and place RSDS/CRPS, Fibromyalgia and related conditions into remission.

PERIPHERAL NEUROPATHY STUDY

Patient Summary:

- Peripheral neuropathy is a diagnosis made when patients demonstrate a malfunction of nerve fibers connecting the central nervous system (the brain and spinal cord) and the rest of the body.
- This may involve just one particular nerve or it may involve many nerve fibers at the same time.
- When only one nerve fiber section is involved, the patient may experience numbness or pain, in one area of their body.
- Many times when there are multiple nerves involved, the area of numbness or pain will appear as a "stocking" or "glove" distribution.
- Peripheral neuropathies may be inherited, caused by other diseases such as diabetes, or may be the result of injury.
- No matter what the cause, the end result is that the peripheral nerve no longer is able to conduct its messages in a normal manner.
- Research has shown that this is due to a lack of adequate oxygen being supplied to the nerve. It has been demonstrated in the laboratory that peripheral neuropathies can be reversed, by supplying adequate oxygen to the nerves.
- In our study, we showed that not only did the patients feel better but also that the peripheral neuropathies could be improved with our treatments. 59% of the patients who received one hour of treatment per day had nerve conduction improvement by the end of one month.

Physician Summary:

- Clinical experience has shown that STS treatments are extremely effective in decreasing the morbidity of Peripheral Neuropathies.
- This is probably due to an increase of endoneural circulation caused by the creation of VIP (Vasoactive Intestinal Polypeptide), CGRP (Calcitonin Gene-related Peptide), and the electrical stimulation itself.
- Multiple digital skin temperature, skin temperature gradients, and photoplethysmography all show that STS treatments increase peripheral perfusion.
- In addition, it has been shown that plasma VIP levels are increased and that heart rate variability decreases, with STS treatments.
- Below, there is a study of STS treatments for peripheral neuropathy patients. 59% of the patients who received one hour of treatment per day had nerve conduction improvement by the end of one month. This included two patients who had not had F waves in tested nerves for over 10 years. Following 30 days of treatment, F waves were detected in these patients.

Effects of Sympathetic Therapy on Chronic Pain and Nerve Conduction Deficits in Peripheral Neuropathy Patients

Abstract. 20 patients suffering from chronic pain, primarily caused by peripheral neuropathies, received sympathetic therapy treatments (Dynatron STS, Dynatronics Corporation, Salt Lake City, Utah). Sympathetic therapy treats the sympathetic nervous system utilizing electric current. Patients, ranging in age from 37 to 75 years old, were treated daily for a period of 28 days. Pre and post nerve conduction velocity testing was performed on 18 of these patients. At the onset of the study, 75% of the patients reported moderate to severe pain. By day five, 50% reported moderate to severe pain. By day eighteen, only 14% of the patients reported moderate to severe pain. At the end of the 28 days, 80% of the patients reported an overall improvement in their quality of life, 80% of the patients reported that they were sleeping better, and 40% of the patients were able to significantly reduce their medications (neurontin, ultram, narcotics, etc.). In addition, a majority of the patients had varying degrees of nerve conduction normalization. These patients had previously been unresponsive to other therapeutic regimens.

INTRODUCTION

It is estimated that there are more than 20 million people in the United States who have been diagnosed as having peripheral neuropathies. In the past, physicians have not had an effective treatment for this disease process.

Recently, encouraging results have been seen in the treatment of patients with peripheral neuropathies utilizing the Dynatron STS. This system utilizes low frequency, high intensity transcutaneous sinusoidal waveform stimulation through extremely long sections of specific peripheral nerves, involving specific dermatomes and thermatomes, as well as specific electrode placements. In addition, beat frequencies are chosen to maximize the production of various neuropeptides and neurotransmitters. This combination is formatted to have the stimulation involve the specific pad placement, peripheral nerve pathways, spinal anatomy, sympathetic nervous system anatomy, spinal nerve anatomy, as well as the cellular and tissue physiology so as to benefit the affected areas of the body.

METHODOLOGY

The study was comprised of 20 patients. The patients had a nerve conduction evaluation before and after the 28 days of treatment. The patients were not allowed to miss more than 2 days in a row nor more than a total of 3 days throughout the 28 days of treatment. The patients were not allowed to have skin piercing procedures (injections or surgery) during the study. Due to a lack of communication between medical offices, two of the patients did not receive pre-treatment nerve conduction studies. Therefore, the subjective summary is for 20 patients but the objective summary is only for 18 patients.

The patients completed a pain grid depicting the area of worst pain, as well as secondary areas of pain. The pad placement protocols were chosen from the Dynatronic STS clinical software, on the basis of the location of the worst pain, that day. The patients received a total of one hour of treatment, per day. The treatment was divided into a 20 minute and 40 minute section. Treatment was given through the hands and the feet. If the patient's worst pain was above the waist, the 40-minute treatment was given through the hands and the 20-minute treatment was given through the feet. If the patient's worst pain was below the waist, the 40-minute treatment was given through the feet and the 20-minute treatment was given through the hands.

RESULTS

SUBJECTIVE (20 PATIENTS):

85% (17) reported at least 45% relief of all symptoms

10% (2) reported between 35 and 45% relief of all symptoms

5% (1) did not report pain relief but did report other improvements.

40% (8) were able to significantly reduce their medications (neurontin, ultram, and narcotics)

80% (16) reported an overall improvement in their quality of life

80% (16) reported better sleep

85% (17) stated that they wished to continue the daily treatments

OBJECTIVE (18 PATIENTS):

Overall, 59% (11) of the patients had improvement in their nerve conduction.

22% (4) had nerve conduction when there had been no conduction prior to the study

5% (1) had an "F" wave when none was apparent prior to the study

27% (5) had improvement in the "F" wave

27% (5) had CMAP amplitude improvement

27% (5) had Motor Conduction Velocity improvement

5% (1) had Motor Distal Latency improvement

DISCUSSION

It has been shown by numerous investigators that a reduction or impaired blood flow and the resultant endoneurial hypoxia are important factors underlying nerve conduction deficits. Cameron showed that nerve blood flow in chronic experimental diabetes was reduced by 41% as early as 1 week after diabetes induction. However, with a chemical adrenergic sympathectomy, blood flow increased to within the normal range. Conduction velocity, depressed by 26% with diabetes, was normalized by treatment. (3)

Other authors report similar results. Terata found that in 4-week, streptozotocin-induced diabetic rats, the sciatic motor nerve conduction velocity was decreased by 22% and the sciatic endoneural blood flow was decreased by 49%. (23)

Cameron also reported that chronic increases in nerve electrical activation promote mechanisms that reverse conduction deficits in diabetic rats. (4)

In another paper Cameron concluded that electrical stimulation causes activity-related improvements in diabetic nerve blood flow and metabolism. He felt that the data demonstrated that chronic electrical activation of one sciatic nerve branch can, over several days, produce profound changes in conduction velocity that also affects axons not directly stimulated but that share the same sciatic vasa nervorum blood supply and microenvironment. Sciatic endoneurial blood flow is reduced by diabetes and the consequent endoneurial hypoxia has been hypothesized to result in short-term changes because of reduced ATP production and long-term damage to axons and Schwann cells mediated by oxygen-free radicals. (5)

Winter postulated that there is an obvious decrease in electrical transmission along the nerves that are pathologically changed by demyelinization, which delays or completely interrupts nerve signals. The electrical deficit blocking the polarization and depolarization to take place can be normalized by the biphasic square wave supplied by TNS. (25)

Brain found that a subcutaneous injection of VIP induces a local erythema persisting for 3 hours. In contrast, CGRP induced an intense local erythema, slow in onset but very persistent, up to 10-12 hours duration at high doses. Brain found that in some patients with Raynaud's phenomenon or diabetic polyneuropathy, electrical transcutaneous nerve stimulation induces vasodilation and relief from ischemic pain. It has been suggested that the release of an endogenous vasodilator is partly responsible for the beneficial effects. Transcutaneous nerve stimulation has been associated with a rise in plasma VIP in these patients and normal individuals, although further studies have suggested that this endogenous vasodilator is not VIP but is probably CGRP. In the periphery, immunoreactive CGRP was found in thin beaded nerve fibers that were associated with the smooth muscle of blood vessels and was found to work on arterioles. (1)

Jager found that skin blood flow, assessed by a laser Doppler unit, was increased up to 682% of the basal level by CGRP. CGRP increased regional blood flow to the brain and the skin at the expense of the gastrointestinal tract. (9)

Kaada found that distant, low frequency TNS (2 Hz) improved microcirculation in ischemic limbs of patients with Raynaud's phenomenon and diabetic neuropathy and to accelerate healing of chronic skin ulcerations.

He also found that skin temperature increased 1.8 to 2.8 degrees centigrade and persisted for several hours after treatment. Plasma VIP was increased 60% following stimulation.

Kaada felt that the improved microcirculation of the skin was most likely caused by a sympatho-inhibition effectuated through a central serotoninergic link, since the response was blocked by the serotonin blocker cyproheptadine. In addition, the vasodilation was proportional to the increase in plasma VIP.

He stated that the mechanism of the relief of pain from wounds and ulcers was probably due to the vasodilation and endorphins, as well as the release of ACTH and adrenocortical hormones caused by the TNS. Naloxone did not alter the vasodilatory effect or pain relief. He felt that this was due to an increase in VIP, which evidently affects the arterio-venous anastomoses. (12)(13)(14)

Kaada felt that the primary cause of the improved microcirculation resulting from the electrical stimulation may be due to:

1. Sympatho-inhibition. It has been shown that this reflex inhibition is relayed over the depressor area of the medulla oblongata. Experiments have shown that the vasodilatory response can be antagonized by the administration of a central serotonin blocker, suggesting the involvement of a central serotonergic link.

2. Release of a vasodilatory substance. Probably vasoactive intestinal polypeptide.

3. ACTH-release. In addition to improved microcirculation, tissue repair may possibly also be accelerated by an endogenous ACTH-release which has been shown to occur in response to low-frequency peripheral stimulation. (10)

VIP is not a blood-borne hormone. An increase in plasma VIP in the systemic circulation represents an overflow from synapses, caused either by an increased release or by a reduced degradation of the neuromodulator.

An unexpected finding in these studies was that the resting values of plasma VIP were significantly (about 30%) lower in Raynaud and sclerodermic patients than in normal subjects. It has previously been suggested that one explanation could be that this lower plasma VIP concentration represents a defect in the VIP system in these patients and that it is a pathogenetic factor in the disease. (11)

Said states that VIP stimulates the release of multiple chemicals, including serotonin. It has been shown that VIP enhances the binding of serotonin to its receptors in rat hippocampus.

VIP binding sites have been identified in the hypothalamus, cerebral cortex, and pineal. Intracerebroventricular administration of VIP has a hypnogenic effect in rats and cats rendered partially insomniac. VIP stimulates cyclic AMP production, which in turn increases the production of melatonin.

VIP is a dominant factor in increasing the availability of glucose from glycogen, promotes glucose utilization, and inhibits platelet aggregation. (6)(20)

The concentration of (VIP) in CSF from diabetic patients was significantly decreased compared with that from the controls. (24)

It has been found that diabetic patients without clinical or neurophysiological evidence of polyneuropathy had reduced density of CGRP fibers when compared to controls. (17)

It was found that CGRP retains biological activity for long periods in cutaneous tissue fluid. Even extremely small amounts of substance P converts the longlasting vasodilation induced by CGRP into a transient response. It was found that substance P causes a release of proteolytic enzymes from mast cells, which cause the destruction of CGRP. (2)

It has been found that CGRP induces a rapid and dose-dependent accumulation of intracellular cyclic AMP(cAMP). CGRP synthesis is increased after nerve injury, suggesting that this peptide may play a role in nerve regeneration. CGRP promotes Schwann cell proliferation through an activation of certain c-AMP pathways. (19)

There was a significant increase in intracellular cAMP with low-frequency (10 Hz) currents. (16)(22)

It was found that VIP caused increased intracellular cAMP. (18)

Yamamoto showed that there is a c-AMP-dependent differential regulation of Schwann cell extracellular matrix gene expression, which may be related to the role of each ECM molecule in the peripheral nerve development and regeneration. (26)

It was found that the cyclic AMP (cAMP) content in the sciatic nerves of diabetic rats was significantly lower than in those of normal rats. Administration of dibutyryl cyclic AMP significantly restored the cAMP content in the sciatic nerves and motor nerve conduction velocity, which reflects nerve function.

It was concluded that reduction of cAMP content in peripheral nerves may be involved in the pathogenesis of diabetic neuropathy and is mainly caused by the impairment of adenylate cyclase activity in the diabetic state. (21)

Existing data indicates that F-wave studies are the most sensitive measure of nerve pathology, with the least day-to-day variability. (7)(8)(15)

CONCLUSIONS

In reviewing this study's results, it could be hypothesized that improved circulation to the nerves resulted in the improvement in the peripheral neuropathy patients. The current working hypothesis for this study is that the STS treatments are effective due to a combination of the following aspects of the treatments: low frequency electrical current passing through long sections of nerves, production of cyclic adenosine monophosphate, electrode pad placement (including acupuncture points), the choice of the peripheral nerves being stimulated so that there is a cross-over effect in the CNS, leakage of action potentials from the nerves being stimulated into nerves entering the sympathetic ganglia, the quadrilateral location of stimulation, creation of action potentials through sympathetic nerves in the peripheral nerves being stimulated, production of ACTH, production of dynorphins, enkephalins or beta-endorphins, creation of action potentials through sympathetic nerves in the peripheral nerves being stimulated which enter the sympathetic ganglia directly, local analgesia resulting in a decrease of substance P; and/or the production of circulation altering neuropeptides such as vasoactive intestinal polypeptide (VIP) and calcitonin gene-related peptide (CGRP).

The patients in this study were able to improve subjectively in spite of a reduction of medications. In addition, this study showed that the Dynatron STS System was able to improve the nerve conduction in a significant portion of the patients. Most impressive of the follow up testing was that 32% of the patients tested had improvement in the F-wave studies.

REFERENCES

These are early studies that put me on a path of understanding the basic premises I needed to know to in order to develop the treatments I use today.

1   Brain SD, Tippins JR, Morris HR, MacIntyre I, Williams TJ "Potent Vasodilator activity of calcitonin gene-related peptide in human skin" J Invest Dermatol. 1986 Oct;87(4):533-6.

2   Brain SD, Williams TJ. "Substance P regulates the vasodilator activity of calcitonin gene-related peptide." Nature Vol 335 Sept. 1988 3-5.

3   Cameron NE, Cotter MA, Low PA "Nerve blood flow in early experimental diabetes in rats: relation to conduction deficits" Am J Physiol. 1991 Jul;261(1 Pt 1):E1-8.

4   Cameron NE, Cotter MA, Robertson S "Chronic low frequency electrical activation for one week corrects nerve conduction velocity deficits in rats with diabetes of three months duration" Diabetologia. 1989 Oct;32(10):759-61.

5   Cameron NE, Cotter MA, Robertson S, Maxfield EK "Nerve function in experimental diabetes in rats: effects of electrical stimulation" Am J Physiol. 1993 Feb;264(2 Pt 1):E161-6.

6   Fahrenkrug J, Emson PC. "Vasoactive intestinal polypeptide: functional aspects." Br Med Bull 1982 Sep;38(3):265-70.

7   Fisher, M.A. "The contemporary role of F-wave studies." Muscle&Nerve 8/97; 1098-1101.

8   Henning A., Stalberg E.,Falck, B. "F-wave latency, the most sensitive nerve conduction parameter in patients with diabetes mellitus." Muscle&Nerve 10/97; 1296-1302.

9   Jager K, Muench R, Seifert H, Beglinger C, Bollinger A, Fischer JA "Calcitonin gene-related peptide (CGRP) causes redistribution of blood flow in humans." Eur J Clin Pharmacol. 1990;39(5):491-4.

10   Kaada B."Promoted healing of chronic ulceration by transcutaneous nerve stimulation (TNS)." Vasa 1983;12(3):262-9.

11   Kaada B. "Successful treatment of esophageal dysmotility and Raynaud's phenomenon in systemic sclerosis and achalasia by transcutaneous nerve stimulation." Scand J Gastroenterol 1987 Nov; 22(9):1137-46.

12   Kaada B. "Systemic sclerosis: successful treatment of ulcerations, pain, Raynaud's phenomenon, calcinosis, and dysphagia by transcutaneous nerve stimulation." Acupunct Electrother Res 1984;9(1):31-44.

13   Kaada B."Vasodilation induced by transcutaneous nerve stimulation in peripheral ischemia (Raynaud's phenomenon and diabetic polyneuropathy." Eur Heart J 1982 Aug;3(4):303-14.

14   Kaada B., Lygren I."Lower plasma levels of some gastrointestinal peptides in Raynaud's disease. Influence of transcutaneous nerve stimulation." Gen Pharmacol 1985;16(2):153-6.

15   Kohara N, Kimura J, Kaji R, Goto Y, Ishii J. "Inter-trial variability of nerve conduction studies, multicenter analysis." Electroencephalogr Clin Neurophysiol 1995; 97:566.

16   Knedlitschek G, Noszvai-Nagy M, Meyer-Waarden H, Schimmelpfeng J, Weibezahn KF, Dertinger H. "Cyclic AMP response in cells exposed to electric fields of different frequencies and intensities." Radiat Environ Biophys 1994; 33(2): 141-7.

17   Lindberger M, Schroder HD, Schultzberg M, Kristensson K, Persson A, Ostman J, Link H. " Nerve fibre studies in skin biopsies in peripheral neuropathies. I. Immunohistochemical analysis of neuropeptides in diabetes mellitus." J Neurol Sci 1989 Nov; 93(2-3): 289-96.

18   O'Dorisio MS, Wood CL, Wenger GD, Vassalo LM. "Cyclic AMP-dependent protein kinase in Molt 4b lymphoblasts: identification by photoaffinity labeling and activation in intact cells by vasoactive intestinal polypeptide (VIP) and peptide histidine isoleucine (PHI)." J Immunol 1985 Jun;134(6):4078-86.

19   Rossi R, Johansson O."Cutaneous innervation and the role of neuronal peptides in cutaneous inflammation: a minireview." Eur J Dermatol 1998 Jul-Aug;8(5):299-306.

20   Said SI. "Vasoactive intestinal polypeptide (VIP): Current Status." Peptides 1984 Mar-Apr;5(2):143-50.

21   Shindo H, Tawata M, Onaya T. "Reduction of cyclic AMP in the sciatic nerve of rats made diabetic with streptozotocin and the mechanism involved." J Endocrinol 1993 Mar; 136(3): 431-8.

22   Sontag W, Dertinger H. "Response of cytosolic calcium, cyclic AMP, and cyclic GMP in Dimethylsulfoxide-differentiated HL-60 cells to modulated low frequency electric currents." Bioelectromagnetics 1998;19(8):452-8.

23   Terata K, Coppey LJ, Davidson EP, Dunlap JA, Gutterman DD, Yorek MA "Acetylcholine-induced arteriolar dilation is reduced in streptozotocin-induced diabetic rats with motor nerve dysfunction" Br J Pharmacol. 1999 Oct;128(3):837-43.

24 Umeda F, Noda K, Ono H, Chijiiwa Y, Nawata H. "Decreased Vasoactive Intestinal Polypeptide (VIP) Level in Cerebrospinal Fluid from Diabetic Patients with Neuropathy"
Fukuoka Igaku Zasshi 1991 Jan;82(1):17-20.

25 Winter A "The use of Transcutaneous Electrical Stimulation (TNS) in the Treatment of Multiple Sclerosis." Journal of Neurosurgical Nursing. December. Vol. 8, No. 2.

26 Yamamoto M, Sobue G, Li M, Mitsuma T, Kimata K, Yamada Y. "cAMP-dependent differential regulation of extracellular matrix (ECM) gene expression in cultured rat Schwann cells." Brain Res 1994 Aug 8; 653(1-2): 335-9.

APPENDIX

The following list describes ten different levels of pain. This guide is given to patients to help them evaluate their pain rate every day before and after treatment. The next sheets ask further information about pain and discomfort locations and levels. On the diagram of the body, patients use colored markers to indicate the areas and intensity of their pain.

RATE YOUR PAIN

0-Pain Free

1-Very minor annoyance-mild aches to some parts of the body. No pain medication needed.

2-Minor annoyance-dull aches to some parts of the body. No pain medication needed.

3-Annoying enough to be distracting. Over-the-counter pain relievers (such as Naproxen Sodium, Acetaminophen, or topical treatments such as Absorbine or Arthritis Pain Relieving rubs) take care of it.

4-Can be ignored if you are really involved in your work, but still distracting. Over-the-counter pain relievers remove pain for 3-4 hours.

5-Can't be ignored for more than 30 minutes. Over-the-counter pain relievers help somewhat (bring pain level 5 to 3 or 4) for 3-4 hours.

6-Can't be ignored for any length of time, but you can still go to work and participate in social activities. Stronger pain killers (such as Ultram) relieve pain for 3-4 hours.

7-Makes it difficult to concentrate, interferes with sleep. You can still function with effort. Stronger pain killers (such as Ultram) only partially effective. (Stronger painkillers bring pain from 7 to 4-6).

8-Physical activity severely limited. You can read and converse with effort. Stronger painkillers (such as Ultram) are not effective. (Narcotic pain killers do bring this pain down to a level 3 or lower).

9-Non-funcional for all practical purposes. Cannot concentrate. Physical activity halted. Panic sets in. (Narcotic painkillers bring the pain level from 9 to the 4-6 level).

10-Totally non-functional. Unable to speak. Crying and/or moaning uncontrollably. Near delirium.

Patient STS Key

In order to better treat your pain, please check the symptoms that apply and indicate the severity of your symptoms below.

SCALE: 0 = None   10 = Extremely Severe

———————   Indigestion   ———————   (0- 10)

———————   Nausea   ———————   (0- 10)

———————   Diarrhea   ———————   (0- 10)

———————   Constipation   ——————— (0- 10)

———————   Menstrual Cramps   ———————   (0- 10)

———————   Headache   ———————   (0- 10)

———————   Cold or Flu   ———————   (0- 10)

———————   Allergies   ———————   (0- 10)

———————   Asthma   ———————   (0- 10)

———————   Joint Pain ———————   (0- 10) ____FINGERS____ELBOW____SHOULDER____NECK
                                            ____BACK____HIP ____KNEE____ANKLE___TOES

———————   Generalized Fatigue   ———————   (0- 10)

———————   Memory Problems   ———————   (0- 10)

———————   Knee Pain   ———————   (0- 10)

MEDICATIONS: Please list the name of all medications, the strength, and how often during the past 24- hour day you take them (please state if any have been reduced or increased, since the last treatment).

_____

_____

_____

_____

_____

_____

Following yesterday's treatment, what was the highest symptom relief that you experienced?

No Relief   Slight Relief   Some Relief   Good Relief   Complete Relief

How long did symptom relief last?

Less than 1 hour   1-4 hours   4-7 hours   7-10 hours   10+ hours

Please rate you average symptom severity level for the previous 24 hours. 0 = none – 10 = severe

0   1   2   3   4   5   6   7   8   9   10

Compared to yesterday, please rate today's level of symptom severity.

Much Worse   Worse   About the Same   Better   Much Better

Compared to before you began the treatment program, please rate today's level of symptom severity?

Much Worse   Worse   About the Same   Better   Much Better

Please rate your sleep pattern from the previous 24 hrs. Please consider all sleep, including naps.

Less than 2 hours   2-4 hours   4-6 hours   6-8 hours   8 or more hours

Please evaluate how effective you feel the treatment has been, thus far.

Not Effective   Slightly Effective   Effective   Very Effective   Extremely Effective

Please indicate any of your medications you reduced or increase over the past 24 hours.
Please indicate by how much the medication was reduced or increased.

********Please rate the following symptoms on a scale of 0-10******
0 (none)   5 (moderate)   10 (extreme)

Feet

Burning ____ L ____ R	Ankle ____ L ____ R	Fatigue ____	Indigestion ____
Pain ____ L ____ R	Leg ____ L ____ R	Abdomen ____	Insomnia ____
Numbness ____ L ____ R	Knee ____ L ____ R	Neck ____	Nausea ____
Tingling ____ L ____ R	Hip ____ L ____ R	Head ____	Constipation ____
Discoloration ____ L ____ R	Arm ____ L ____ R	Chest ____	Diarrhea ____
Swelling ____ L ____ R	Elbow ____ L ____ R	Jaw/Face ____	Memory Problems ____
Aching ____ L ____ R	Hand ____ L ____ R	Upper Back ____	Dizzy / Lightheadedness ____
Itching ____ L ____ R	Wrist ____ L ____ R	Mid Back ____	Mood Swings ____
Stiffness ____ L ____ R	Shoulder ____ L ____ R	Lower Back ____	Total ____ / 530

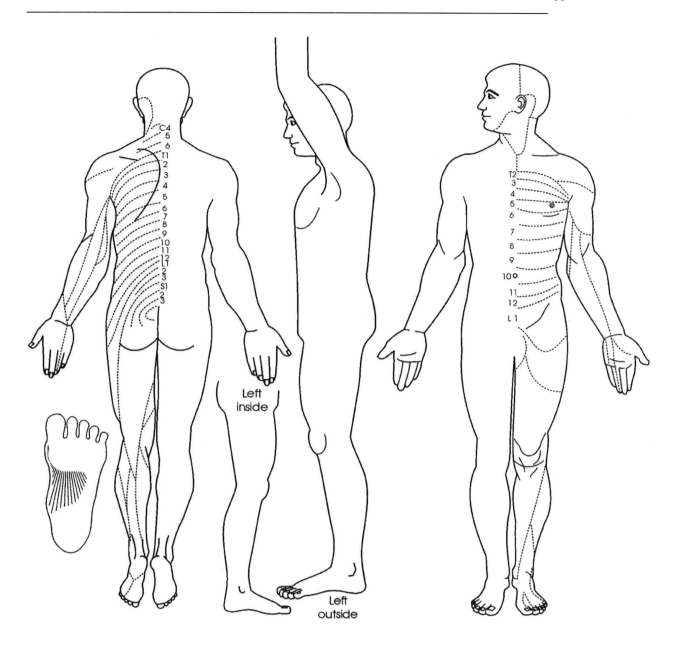

Every day in the clinic, patients use this sheet and colored markers to highlight their areas of pain.

□

4120434

Made in the USA
Charleston, SC
02 December 2009